POW/MIA AMERICA'S MISSING MEN

The Men We Left Behind

CHIMP ROBERTSON

POW/MIA AMERICA'S MISSING MEN

The Men We Left Behind

CHIMP ROBERTSON

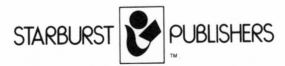

STARBURST PUBLISHERS

P.O. Box 4123, Lancaster, Pennsylvania 17604

To schedule Author appearances write:
Author Appearances, Starburst Promotions, P.O. Box 4123
Lancaster, Pennsylvania 17604 or call (717) 293-0939

Credits:
POW photos courtesy Department of Defense
POW/MIA logo courtesy National League of Families of
    American Prisoners and Missing in Southeast Asia

First Printing, October 1995

ISBN: 0-914984-64-0
Library of Congress Catalog Number 94-66614
Printed in the United States of America

Dedication

For *Ruby*, my Mother
and the memory of my dad, *Alton T. Robertson, Sr.*, a
Texas Panhandle Cowboy and Veteran of World War II,
and in memory of my wife, *Donna*, a
gallant warrior in her own right, who
fought the battle against cancer,
and our children,
Bryan, Gary, Todd, Jill and *Brian*.

There have been many books written on Vietnam. Most of those books focused on a specific battle, a special heroic effort or a certain member of the Armed Forces who went beyond the call of duty.

This book is dedicated to the American POW/MIAs from all wars. As sad as it is, the U.S. government's most recent POW/MIA statistics list 1,250 from World War I, 78,751 from World War II, 8,177 from Korea and 2,266 from Vietnam.

Also, I dedicate this book to the families and loved ones of all POW/MIAs, especially to those gallant American servicemen and women who have answered the last roll call so you and I could continue to live in freedom in America.

Finally, I dedicate it to the brave Americans who answered the call of their country, went to war in Southeast Asia, and "did come back."

In the words of Sgt. Dan Lewis of the 25th Infantry, "God bless us all."

Chimp Robertson,
Tahlequah, Oklahoma

Acknowledgments

Many people deserve thanks for the help and encouragement they gave me during the development of this book. This project received assistance from many who contributed to the information within and I wish to thank them all.

I especially want to acknowledge all the veterans who shared their thoughts, experiences and first-hand recollections and spent their valuable time writing and sending me their responses.

A very special thanks goes to Ann Mills Griffiths, Executive Director and Mary C. Backley, Director of Operations of the National League of Families of American Prisoners and Missing in Southeast Asia.

And, thanks to Mr. Miles Z. Epstein, Associate Editor and Mr. John F. Sommer, Jr., Executive Director of *The American Legion* magazine and to Mr. Gary L. Bloomfield, Managing Editor/Assistant Director of *VFW* magazine.

Also, the *Pride Of Tulsa Vietnam Veterans of America Chapter Newsletter*, Kathleen Aris, *Wallkill Valley Times*, and the Department of Defense. Their assistance was invaluable.

Photos of POWs were made available by Mr. Ken Carter of the Department of Defense, Washington, D.C. To him I owe a special debt of gratitude.

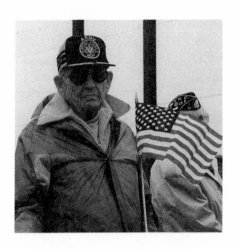

Special Tribute

Col. James D. Ogletree has seen it all. He was born in 1905 in Gruene, Texas, the town his grandfather founded. He graduated from Texas A&M and was commissioned by ROTC as a second lieutenant. He worked for the Civilian Conservation Corp. (CCC) until he was called to active service at Ft. Sill, Oklahoma in 1940.

He was promoted to Captain and sent to a new outfit called the Tank Destroyers at Ft. Carson, Colorado, then to Ft. Hood, Texas. Gen. Dwight D. Eisehower said the "Tank Destroyers" were worth their weight in gold.

Ogletree went overseas as Battery Commander of the 564th Field Artillery Battalion in the 71st Infantry Division assigned to Gen. Patton's Third Army.

Having landed at La Havre, France, they took over the walled town of Bitche on the German-French border and replaced the battle-weary 100th Division.

Crossing the Rhine River at Oppenheim on Easter night, they reached the industrial city of Meiningen. They kept up the push until they came to Steyer, Austria. On May 2, 1945, they got orders to cease fire. The war was over. Ogletree's division stayed in Germany as part of the "Occupation Forces" until March, 1947.

Colonel Ogletree was made Major and joined Gen. I. D. White's occupation constabulary. Ogletree's last assignment was as Group Commander of the 2nd QM Group in the 7th Army in Germany under Gen. Bruce Clark, the Hero of the Battle of the Bulge. Ogletree retired July 31, 1958 as a full Colonel.

He has seen us at our worst and our best. He came with the century. He fought our enemies. He has educated the hope of tomorrow. His times are our times. He answered the call when his country needed him.

Thank you Col. James D. Ogletree.

Chimp Robertson

Quotes and comments from:

Anderson, William C.
Aris, Kathleen
Armer, William D.
Backley, Mary C.
Bearpaw, Thomas
Beesley, Stanley W.
Benavidez, Roy P. -Sgt.
Bennett, William T. -Gen. Sec.
    Nat. Vietnam Vets Coalition
Bloomfield, Gary L.
Boggs, George Edward
Boren, David -U.S. Senator
Borowski, Alex
Briggs, Leon
Brooks, Mack M. -Lt. Col.
Brown, Leslie L.
Brumbach, Raymond W.
Carney, John F.
Carter, Ken
Cheney, Dick
Christian, Richard
Cook, Joel H.
Crews, John
Culver, William L.
Decker, Carl J.
Duffield, Jimmy
Epstein, Miles
Forrester, Larry D.
Fortune, David Edward
Gillotte, Tony -New York Journalist
Gore, Al -Vice President
Griffiths, Ann Mills
Guthrie, Bennett Jr.
Hamilton, Donovan
Hannah, Dennis
Henry, Warren B.
Horner, Charles "Chief"
Hrdlicka, Carol
Kerry, John F. -Senator
Ketcher, John A.
Koch, George
Lanning, Michael Lee
Leppelman, John L. (Lepp)
Lewis, Dan
Locke, Archie
Lugar, Richard -Senator
Maddex, Vince
Marks, Robert L.
McCaffery, Barry R. -Gen.
McCain, John -Senator
McDaniel, Eugene "Red" -Capt.
Mooney, Jerry -Sgt. USAF (Ret.)

Munson, Roger A.
Nickles, Don -Senator
Nordin, Cletys
Norris, Robert
North, Oliver
Ogletree, James -Col.
Oldfield, Barney
Olson, Leif Robert
Payne, Paul B.
Peck, Millard A. -Col. USA (Ret.)
Penny, Douglass W.
Perry Dwight
Peterson, Glenn E.
Plimpton, George
Pribram, John G,
Reichart, Carl T.
Reid, John III
Risner, Robinson "Robbie" -Gen.
Rockholt, Eugene
Rusk, Dean
Rutledge, Lee
Salisbury, Harrison E.
Scott, Robert
Smith, Bob -Senator
Smith, James P. (Jim)
Sommer, John F. Jr.
Sparks, Oscar S.
Starr, Jerold M.
Swanson, Raymond Q.
Taylor, Thomas H.
Tighe, Eugene -Lt. Gen. USAF (Ret.)
Vardeman, William S. (Bill)
Vessey, John W. Jr. -Gen. USA (Ret.)
Wagner, James R.
Waylett, Lillis L. (Monte)
Weaver, Jim
Weese, Don -State Representative
Weidner, Bill
Westmoreland, William C. -Gen.
Wilson, Hubert E.
Zotter, Charles C.
Zumwalt, E.R. Jr. -Adm. USN (Ret.)
The American Legion magazine
Department of the Army
Department of Veteran Affairs
National League of Families of
    Missing Americans
POW/MIA News
Pride of Tulsa Vietnam Veterans
VFW magazine
Walkill Valley Times

Selected Comments

"Many thanks for your hard work and research into the issue of our American POWs and MIAs."

Oliver North, U.S. Army Veteran, author and politician

"A must-read for every American who is interested in the servicemen and women—in the past and in the future."

William Anderson, screenwriter and author of *Bat-21,*
22-year USAF Veteran

"I believe in this book. Chimp Robertson has pointed out clearly: 'Our job is not yet done.'"

Dale Robertson, Hollywood movie actor, W.W. II Veteran

"Chimp Robertson has put on paper a most captivating and compelling collection of facts and information about a 'war' that most Americans have chosen to ignore. Chimp has painfully stirred old memories and reignited the passions of loyalty and self-preservation. Chimp very effectively points out that, in our open society, too much secrecy surrounds the records of those who, in good and honorable faith in their country and government, remain unaccounted for after nearly 20 years. This raises legitimate questions: What is being covered up or hidden? Who is being protected?"

John R. deSteiguer, Exec. Dir.-Oklahoma Schools Advisory Council,
24-year Navy veteran

"*POW/MIA–America's Missing Men* is riveting and relevant to a number of issues our country is still facing. I offer you best wishes for what will certainly be inspirational for those who read it."

Jack Mildren, Oklahoma Lieutenant Governor

". . .(*POW/MIA–America's Missing Men*) is outstanding. You are a man very worthy of the recognition you receive for aiding veterans. We, as the Military Order of the Purple Heart, wholeheartedly endorse your book."

Jack Hayes, 1993-94 Oklahoma State Commander of the
Military Order of the Purple Heart

"Chimp Robertson's book, *POW/MIA–America's Missing Men,* is so different because, while it is a useful reference work, it has a strong spiritual concern for the pain connected with this topic. I found the collection of photographs of POW/MIAs to be particularly poignant and informative. The ordinary reader should be fascinated; scholars will learn much. *POW/MIA–America's Missing Men* should be in every public library and university collection . . . (No other author) assembles the treasure trove of facts to be found in Robertson's reverent study."

Peter C. Rollins, Vietnam Veteran, author of 10 books, Regents Professor of
English and American/Film Studies, Oklahoma State University

Contents

Preface

The roots of this book go back to World War II when my Dad was drafted. The separation made me realize how much a family is torn apart when a loved one is taken away to war.

I will never forget the little 45 rpm record Dad sent us from overseas. I can't recall what he said to the others, but when he was talking directly to me, I couldn't hold back the tears. I was nine years old at the time.

Seeing Dad in uniform, and having him come home safely, always made me want to be a soldier. I turned 18 on the 23rd of August, the day the American POWs were coming through the gates of Freedom Village in Korea. That's as close as I came to fighting for my country.

But, I joined the Army anyway, and also served six years in the Texas National Guard. Like many other Americans, I thought there would never be another war.

Then, Vietnam. However, by that time I was too old for the draft, had two children, and was running a 10,000-acre farm and ranch operation. I missed that war too. But, it struck home one day when I was driving down the street and met a friend who was on leave from the Marine Corps.

I hadn't seen him since he had been home and I could tell he was feeling down. I told him I was on my way to a rodeo and asked if he'd like to go along. He thought that was a great idea so we agreed to meet there in one hour.

When I came back, he was there all right, but he was feeling even more down than before. I asked, "What's the matter Bobby?" He said, "Well, I sure want to go to the rodeo with you like we used to, but you see, I leave for Vietnam tomorrow, and I'm wondering if I should go with you or go home."

I said, "Bobby, please, go straight home and spend this last night with your Mom and Dad. That is the most important thing in the world for you to do right now. Don't even think about going with me. Go home."

He did go home, and he did go to Vietnam, but he never came back.

This book was written especially for the thousands like Bobby, who never came back.

Foreword

The author is a proud American patriot and a veteran in the service of his country. He has never been in combat and he has never spent a single day as a prisoner of war in a foreign land. Yet, he has an understanding of the plight of the prisoner of war that is generally only seen in someone who has endured the suffering of that situation.

I was first introduced to this energetic man during his efforts to organize the first annual Oklahoma Veterans Appreciation Banquet, a gala to honor the sacrifices of my home state's veterans.

His untiring devotion to this monumental task has seen it grow into a statewide celebration for our veterans from all branches of service and all our nation's conflicts. It is with this same effort he has attacked the compelling subject of his book, *POW/MIA–America's Missing Men.*

As a young and confident U.S. Marine Harrier Pilot during Operation Desert Storm, I was forced to face my greatest fear as a combat aviator. On January 28, 1991, while flying my seventh mission, my jet was crippled by an Iraqi surface-to-air missile which forced me to eject over enemy held territory. On the ground, I was quickly captured and spent the next 37 days as a prisoner of war in Baghdad, Iraq.

While being held prisoner, my overriding concern was my family having to endure the same tragic uncertainty as those families of the men listed as Missing in Action in Vietnam. For more than two decades those families have painfully contemplated the ultimate fate of their loved ones.

During the Persian Gulf War, every night as the bombs and missiles rained down on Baghdad, I took some comfort knowing my country was still doing something to hasten the end of the war and return my fellow prisoners of war and me to our anxious families.

We, as Desert Storm prisoners of war, in great part, owe our lives to the lessons learned by our predecessors. The lessons taught at the Armed Forces' Survival, Evasion, Resistance and Escape schools, came from their years of suffering. The Code of Conduct they forged through experience helped us maintain our dignity during those trying times and return home with honor. When we as military members sign a formal contract with the U.S. government to defend freedom and democracy, we also expect we are entering an equally binding unwritten contract with the American people.

Military men and women should rightfully expect that if we are willing to die in defense of the ideals of our country, our families can be assured our bodies will be returned with honor to the soil of a grateful nation.

If captured, our countrymen will do everything possible to secure the earliest possible repatriation. Further, that if while being held prisoner, we suffer abuses attempting to comply with the guidelines of the Code of Conduct, the American people will not rest until the perpetrators are held accountable for their actions.

Finally, if listed as Missing in Action, our mighty nation would leave no stone unturned attempting to determine our fate.

However, in Vietnam and Korea, this special unwritten agreement was shamefully broken by our government for political expedience. Fortunately for my generation of veterans, these same people who suffered these injustices vowed not to let history repeat itself.

Since returning from my own ordeal in Southeast Asia, I have had the privilege of talking to many Vietnam prisoners of war about this subject. Some believe they would not have suffered so long in Hanoi had our political leaders committed to keeping sustained pressure on their captors.

In many instances, after devastating airstrikes in and around Hanoi, the prisoners' treatment and living conditions would temporarily improve as the North Vietnamese believed the United States had finally decided to commit to winning the war.

Unfortunately, the same government that needlessly prolonged our prisoners' suffering, also failed in its responsibility to demand the fullest possible accounting of our missing countrymen.

When you read this book, I hope it stirs your emotions as it did mine. Having experienced the harshness of life as a prisoner of war for only 37 days, I now have but a small idea of what those heroic veterans had to endure for years on end.

Whether or not there are still American servicemen alive in Southeast Asia will probably never be known, but as long as there is even the slightest possibility, we owe it to them and their families to aggressively pursue the answers to their fate.

Fortunately, there have always been proud Americans like Mr. Robertson who respect the sacrifices of our country's combat veterans and strive to ensure his fellow Americans don't forget their responsibilities of that unwritten contract.

Capt. Michael Craig Berryman
USMC Desert Storm POW

Part 1

I lift up my eyes to the hills;
from where is my help to come?

Psalms: 121:1

Vietnam Cry

Long, Long ago, in a land of mystery
the young men fought and died; it made history.

Where, oh Where are those young men?
Some have gone on, others weeping,
The rest are in rooms for keeping.

America, America wake up,
Tell the men who run you
to take a look at these young men.
Stop, Listen, hear the cry, the
"Vietnam Cry!"

Too much to explain, to feel, to tell
"Their war" the "Hurting war"
It hit the men right to the core
Their hearts, minds, bodies and souls.
Did they find their friends in the holes?

Many, Many years gone by
Have they forgotten, no glory,
no ribbons, no flags, no pats on the back?
No, Stop, Listen, hear the cry, the
"Vietnam Cry!"

Can't you see, America, what you've done?
The men in high places fall to their faces
The Vietnam Vets fought their war
But they wouldn't trade it for the
laces in high places.

Stop, Listen, hear the Cry, the
Vietnam Cry!

This poem was written for Mr. William Brocker by his wife, Deb

POW/MIAs   **19**

POW/MIAs

"Doubts Are More Cruel Than the Worst of Truths"
Moliére, Le Misanthrope

"I Knew Wherever I Was, You Thought Of Me,
and if I Got in a Tight Place, You Would Come, if Alive"
William Tecumseh Sherman
in a letter to Ulysses S. Grant

What is our duty to our POW/MIAs? What really happened to America's POWs and why? Should we fight to get our men back and fight to expose what was done to keep them POWs? Do you believe there are American POWs still being held against their will in Southeast Asia?

POW/MIAs! What should we know, tell or do about American Fighting Men missing in the Vietnam War? Did we, "the U.S. government," knowingly leave Americans behind when our troops pulled out of Vietnam?

First, we should pray for the persecuted, the prisoners and all who are in danger, that they may be relieved and protected.

Next, we should be very selective where we send young American soldiers and have it clear in our goals and be prepared to win a victory as quickly as possible. Some say the embargo should never be lifted until the POW/MIA issue is settled to America's satisfaction.

Surely there are few things that boost a man's pride more than being part of America's military force. It's so reassuring to know that he will be standing beside some of the world's best trained and equipped fighting men despite the many handicaps such as adverse terrain and weather conditions or possibly overwhelming enemy troops.

In fact, the concern of trying hard and performing well seems to be a preoccupation with USA troops every day of the year and has been since American soldiers were shipped overseas to become part of the Allied Forces during the First World War in 1917 and 1918. So, what do we owe them?

What are some of the most important things to know about our POW/MIAs? Shouldn't we have a full accounting of those still listed as POW/MIA? It could be that there is help for those still missing.

The secrecy that cloaks the POW/MIA issue has led many people to believe that there are some in government who don't want the truth to come out. The natural question is, "Why?"

According to an article in *The American Legion* magazine, the National Commander said, "Nineteen years after President Richard Nixon declared that '. . . all of our courageous prisoners of war (have been) set free and (are) here, back home in America,' 2,267 American families still live in a twilight zone of anxiety and uncertainty. The war is over, but their loved ones have not returned. Their lives are on hold, waiting for answers that may never come. America is at peace, yet they have no peace."

There are many tragic chapters in the Vietnam War. Perhaps, the most tragic of all, the war that the government did not then have the will to win, it does not now have the courage to end honorably. The only way to end it honorably is by insisting on a full accounting of our "missing," before even considering granting full diplomatic recognition to this former enemy.

Seventy-three percent do not believe that Vietnam has honored the one condition set down nearly 20 years ago as a prerequisite of diplomatic recognition.

We do not seek to block the exploration of Vietnam's rich oil deposits. But we do demand that our nation not abandon its honor in order to accomplish these objectives.

No, Vietnam has not dealt with this issue honestly. But I suspect that our government hasn't either.

Vietnam's Communist economy is crumbling and it thirsts for American dollars to survive. If ever there was a time in our history that we could demand and receive a full accounting, it is now. This is what we must do before surrendering the only leverage we have.

While it is time for Vietnam to level with us, it is also time for the U.S. government to level with its own citizens.

In the course of its deliberations, we believe it is time to declassify the millions of documents we have related to our missing and POWs.

It's also appropriate for the Select Committee to investigate charges that individuals within the United States government have intimidated, coerced, discredited and ignored sources who have provided data on living POWs.

It's time for us to admit our own mistakes and commit ourselves to an honest effort to honorably close this chapter in our nation's history.

But, before we normalize, drill for oil, lift our economic embargo, or allow international financial aid—before we do any of this, we must fully account for our "missing" and our prisoners of war.

The United States is moving closer to normalization of relations with Hanoi, despite the failure to get a full accounting of American POW/MIAs. The State Department lifted a ban on U.S.-organized travel to Vietnam, and was prepared to ease up on travel restrictions on Vietnamese diplomats in the United States, before the FBI objected. If the U.S. trade embargo is lifted, veterans groups such as the National Vietnam Veterans Coalition are prepared to boycott U.S. companies that do business with Hanoi.

Some congressmen are expected to strongly press for legislation that would provide foreign aid to the Commonwealth of Independent States, the former Soviet Union, contingent on receiving detailed information about Americans being held against their will there—including Vietnam POWs.

To give Vietnam what it wants now, without a full accounting, would seal the last secrets of the Vietnam War, forever. The price is too high for any nation "under God" to pay.

We believed we would not abandon our men. Yet, the U.S. government's most recent POW/MIA statistics list 2,267 Americans unaccounted for after the Vietnam War. Questions about U.S. POW/MIAs outnumber answers.

At the Pentagon, where rules and regulations are everything, rarely is a powerful high-ranking officer openly challenged by a member of his own staff. But, that is exactly what retired Army Col. Millard A. Peck decided he had to do.

Colonel Peck resigned his post with the Defense Intelligence Agency (DIA) in protest. As chief of DIA's Special Office for Prisoners of War and Missing in Action, his job was to track down 2,267 Americans who are still listed as POW/MIAs from the Vietnam War—to bring every American, dead or alive, home from Southeast Asia.

"I didn't want to be part of a phony effort," Peck told *The American Legion* magazine.

A decorated Vietnam veteran, Peck became convinced that the U.S. government abandoned American servicemen in Southeast Asia. He wasn't the first military officer to reach this conclusion.

In 1981, retired Air Force Lt. Gen. Eugene Tighe, then director of the DIA, testified before Congress that American POWs had been left behind in Southeast Asia.

Nobody listened.

"It's the families of these men who take the worst beating," says Richard Christian of the Legion's Washington office. And he should know. As one of the American Legion's POW/MIA researchers, Christian gets calls on nights and weekends from families who are frustrated.

"These people want to know what happened to their sons, their husbands, their fathers and their brothers," Christian says. "All they get from the Pentagon is a sheet of paper that's all blacked out except for three lines. It's a cold process devoid of compassion."

Christian, accompanied by two editors from *The American Legion* magazine, delivered this message personally to retired Army Gen. John W. Vessey Jr. at his Pentagon Office.

Vessey agreed: "We have the sensitivity of a pile driver in dealing with all of the families," Vessey said as he shook his head, leaned forward, and straightened his necktie.

A former Chairman of the Joint Chiefs of Staff, today Vessey serves as Presidential Emissary to Hanoi for POW/MIA Affairs, a de facto Ambassador to Vietnam on the POW/MIA issue. In a 1988 interview, confirming the findings of Colonel Peck and General Tighe, he said ". . . there is good evidence that there are live prisoners, and it is in the Vietnamese interest to straighten out their relations with the United States."

Today, the Socialist Republic of Vietnam is trying to do just that, normalize relations with the United States of America. And the great fear among many concerned with the POW/MIA issue is that formal ties—establishing diplomatic relations and lifting America's economic embargo on Vietnam—will destroy the last hope of accounting for and recovering America's missing.

"It's a death warrant," says Kathy Borah Duez, a sister of missing Navy pilot Lt. Daniel Borah, Jr. Her brother was shot down over South Vietnam in 1972.

Soldiers who fought on the ground in Vietnam, like Peck, can't help but remember the tactics of the North Vietnamese (NVA) and the Viet Cong (VC). They used the neighboring countries of Laos and Cambodia to sneak into South Vietnam and attack American forces. They would mix with the rural population of the Southern villagers by day and launch attacks by night.

U.S. troops could not tell the difference between friend and enemy. Now, almost 20 years later, America still can't. Time is running out.

While Americans may not want to believe that their country abandoned some of the men it sent to fight the Vietnam War, many believe that is what happened.

Sixty-four percent say that there are still American POWs in Southeast Asia, according to a 1990 Gallup Poll. In a 1991 CNN/*Time* Poll, 70 percent of the American people say that Vietnam is still holding American prisoners.

Torture was common for American prisoners, despite Vietnam's claims of compassionate treatment. Why should we believe they are telling the truth now?

For U.S. companies to gain access to Vietnam's oil, the United States would have to normalize relations with Vietnam within a year, according to an East-West Center report. The U.S. government imposed an economic embargo on Communist Vietnam in 1964 and American companies cannot legally do business there.

According to the East-West Center, Vietnam has the potential to produce between 1.5 billion and 3 billion barrels of oil, worth an estimated $3 billion per year in the next 10 to 15 years.

Sen. Richard Lugar of Indiana said: "The Vietnamese government told me they had set aside some of the prime oil locations for American investment." Lugar recently completed a trip to Vietnam on behalf of the U.S. Senate.

A State Department briefing for veterans groups confirmed that American oil companies are pressing hard for normalization.

"Why does it appear that America is rushing to restore diplomatic relations with Vietnam and not North Korea, where over 8,000 Americans are still POW/MIAs?" asks the Legion's National Commander, Dominic D. DiFrancesco. "Have the Vietnamese been more forthcoming? Or is there something that Vietnam has that North Korea doesn't? How many barrels of cheap oil is one American soldier's life worth?"

"Vietnam has traditionally held back enemy POWs after wars," says John F. Sommer Jr., executive director of the Legion's Washington Office. Sommer served as an Army medic in Southeast Asia during the Vietnam War and was part of a fact-finding group that went to Vietnam and Thailand last summer.

"The road map gives the Vietnamese everything they desire—access to financial aid, new markets and diplomatic ties with the United States—without forcing them to come clean with what they know about American POW/MIAs," Sommer says.

The road map effectively removes all of the U.S. leverage against Vietnam: the embargo, international financial aid and diplomatic recognition.

When a copy of this plan fell into the hands of the American Legion, it was immediately apparent that its execution would have some unfortunate consequences for American POW/MIAs. These include:

- Vietnam is not required to meet any specific conditions on the POW/MIA issue. This deal has been introduced at a time when there are new opportunities to find America's missing men. Changes in what was the Soviet Union, a U.S. POW/MIA office in Hanoi, and a congressional investigation, are America's last opportunities.

- History shows that the Vietnamese cannot be trusted. In its language, the road map relies heavily on Vietnam's honesty. That doesn't give much hope to the families of America's 2,267 POW/MIAs. Those who know the Vietnamese, express despair about America's potential for recovering our missing.

- Unfortunately, the U.S. government's track record on the POW/MIA issue isn't much better than Vietnam's. There is evidence of the following: U.S. government officials didn't take the hunt for POW/MIAs seriously; the government's effort to find POW/MIAs was destined to fail from the beginning; and military secrecy buried the truth about America's missing men—in Pentagon files and on the battlefield.

But, there are new opportunities. The fall of communism in the Soviet Union, followed by the disintegration of the Soviet Union itself, could unlock some of the Vietnam War's last secrets. It could explain what happened to some of America's POW/MIAs.

During the Vietnam War, the Soviet Union sent weapons, military advisers and KGB agents to Southeast Asia. As a close Soviet ally, Vietnam was provided with Moscow's most modern military hardware, including the SAM-2, an anti-aircraft missile.

"By mid-1966, the performance of the SAM was an embarrassment," says historian Robert S. Hopkins III, in a *Los Angeles Times* magazine article on POW/MIAs. In 1965, SAMs were able to shoot down U.S. planes only 5 percent of the time.

Said the *Los Angeles Times* magazine: "Soviet prestige—not to mention the war effort—depended on finding out how American planes were evading the SAMs. The obvious sources of up-to-date American intelligence were the hundreds of American airmen who were literally falling into the arms of Moscow's loyal allies, the North Vietnamese."

To retired Air Force Master Sgt. Jerry Mooney, a National Security Agency (NSA) code-breaker and analyst during the Vietnam War, this is not news. He monitored conversations between the North Vietnamese and their Soviet allies, including discussions about American POWs.

According to Mooney, the KGB and other Soviet military outfits interrogated captured American pilots because they wanted to know how U.S. aircraft were so successfully avoiding Soviet anti-aircraft missiles.

Experts like Sergeant Mooney and General Tighe believe that the Vietnamese may have kept some American prisoners for their technical knowledge. And, in some cases, transported U.S. POWs from Vietnam to the Soviet Union.

Mooney tracked the movement of American POWs in Vietnam, Laos and Cambodia while at NAS.

"Usually, what you heard was a reference that they were being moved to the 'friends,'" Mooney says. "Friends" was the Vietnamese code word for Soviet soldiers or KGB.

"Sometimes, with a stroke of luck, you would not only hear the Vietnamese talking or passing a code, but you would also hear Russian conversations going on in the background, talking about what happened or instructing the Vietnamese what to do," Mooney says.

Today, there are sources in the United States and particularly in Russia, that corroborate Mooney's story.

According to newspaper accounts, Terry Minarcin, a retired Air Force Technical Sergeant who worked for Mooney at NSA, also tracked American POWs en route to the Soviets. Minarcin says that Hanoi shipped 22 Americans to Moscow between December 1977 and January 1978, and that these shipments may have continued into the 1980s.

Information on U.S. POW/MIAs is also surfacing in Russia.

According to the *New York Times*, former KGB Maj. Gen. Oleg D. Kalugin, chief of his organization's intelligence activities in Vietnam from 1975 to 1978, admitted interrogating Americans in Vietnam.

According to another article in the *New York Times*, last year on an Australian Television documentary, a Soviet agent ". . . said he had helped fly two Americans (POWs) to the Soviet Union and that he had seen three other captured servicemen on flights from Vietnam."

Adding fuel to the POW/MIA issue, a Soviet newspaper reported last November that an American POW pilot was transported to the Kazakhstan republic and still lives there. The U.S. State Department says it is investigating this report.

As the United States reorganizes its diplomatic relations with the new independent states that once formed the Soviet Union, there is an opportunity to resolve some of the many POW/MIA cases that have a Soviet connection.

If the U.S. government doesn't investigate the Russian POW/MIA information—now—it could betray 2,267 men who fought for this country in Vietnam.

Another new opportunity to resolve the POW/MIA issue lies in the U.S. POW/MIA office in Hanoi.

Established in July 1991, the office is run by Pentagon staff who support the Presidential Emissary to Hanoi for POW/MIA Affairs, Gen. Vessey.

However, for retired Navy Capt. Eugene "Red" McDaniel, a former POW in Vietnam who served as the Navy/Marine Corps liaison to the

House of Representatives, the office is part of the same bureaucracy that has failed to resolve the POW/MIA issue for almost 20 years.

"I think General Vessey is a victim of a flawed policy," Captain McDainel says. "I think that office is a step toward normalization, and not a serious effort to resolve the POW/MIA issue."

Chaired by Navy Vietnam veteran, Sen. John Kerry of Massachusetts, the Senate has created a select committee to investigate the POW/MIA issue.

This committee is expected to have unprecedented access to classified U.S. documents and information, more than the previous 11 congressional investigations, according to *USA Today*.

Other senators on the committee include former POW John McCain of Arizona, former Marine Charles Robb of Virginia, and Navy veteran Jesse Helms of North Carolina.

"After almost 20 years, time is running out for America's missing men," Sommer says. "This committee represents this country's last chance to aggressively pursue the truth about American POW/MIAs in Southeast Asia."

"The road map needs to take a back seat to all of these new opportunities to resolve the POW/MIA issue—changes in the Soviet Union, the U.S. POW/MIA office in Hanoi and the senate select committee," Sommer says.

Selling POWS! The admission of KGB officials like General Kalugin—namely that they interrogated American POWs in Vietnam and in the Soviet Union—raises a disturbing certainty.

If what they say can be proven, then North Vietnam lied to the United States in 1973 and did not return all of its American POWs. If true, this means that there were in 1973 and could still be captured U.S. servicemen alive in Southeast Asia.

The Vietnamese can't be trusted on the POW/MIA issue. They've proven that.

The U.S. approached Vietnam about normalizing relations two times in the 1970s: in March 1976 and between 1977 and 1978. But the Vietnamese continued to link normalizing relations with receiving financial aid from the United States.

Five days after the signing of the Paris Peace Accords, which ended direct U.S. involvement in the Vietnam War, U.S. Secretary of State Henry Kissinger delivered a letter dated Feburary 1, 1973, promising more than $3 billion in post-war reconstruction aid to the Prime Minister of North Vietnam, according to "An Examination of U.S. Policy Toward POW/MIAs," a 1991 POW/MIA report by the Republican staff of the

Senate Committee on Foreign Relations, commissioned by North Carolina Senator Jesse Helms.

The Vietnamese considered this aid as war reparations from the damage the U.S. military inflicted on their country, according to retired Army Col. John H. Madison, Jr., former chief of the Four Party Joint Military Team between 1974 and 1975.

The Four Party Joint Military Team was a Saigon-based group with the mission of accounting for American MIAs. The team included representatives of the United States, South Vietnam, North Vietnam and the Viet Cong.

But the letter's contents, the promise of financial aid, never made it through Congress and got buried amid the political chaos of Watergate. Vietnam never received financial aid from the United States.

"They are still hanging on to the idea that we are going to give them some money," Colonel Madison says. "When the Four Party Joint Military Team used to go up to Hanoi—we went up there every Friday on a liaison flight in a U.S. Air Force C-130—the North Vietnamese would point out this rail yard on the north side of the Red River.

"It was completely cut out by the B-52s' Christmas raid of 1972. And they told me that 'when you people give us the money to fix this, we might give you some information on your POW/MIAs,'" Madison says.

Observing the harsh treatment of American POWs, the Senate, in an 88–3 roll call vote, voted to "bar any aid to North Vietnam," according to the Associated Press. Many fear that the Vietnamese held on to Americans because they were never paid. After all, selling hostages and POWs is a Vietnamese tradition.

The United States gave the Vietnamese over 5,000 names of POWs. Only 591 were returned. Similarly, the French got back only one-third of the prisoners that it claimed were in the hands of the Vietnamese.

"Certainly, they know a great deal more about POW/MIAs than they've told the United States," Madison says.

Vietnam never returned any POWs who were maimed in any way. General Tighe suspects that this could be yet another reason that some American POWs were not released.

For almost 20 years, the U.S. government's efforts on the POW/MIA issue may have been half-hearted and appear to have been destined to fail. POWs have been seen by five successive administrations as a political liability and virtually ignored. The government, in its zest to cross names off the POW/MIA list, has positively identified remains without sufficient scientific evidence and information about POW/MIAs is so highly classified that the people who could act on it never see it.

In many ways, the 2,267 POW/MIAs in Southeast Asia are a casualty of American Politics.

"To deal with Watergate politically, Richard Nixon and the State Department decided that the POWs were all dead," says McDaniel.

McDaniel believes that the U.S. government knowingly left American POWs behind in Southeast Asia after 1973.

"On April 12, 1973, we declared them all dead," McDaniel says. "That became policy—a flawed policy to deal with Watergate politically."

After Operation Homecoming in 1973, the last release of American POWs by the North Vietnamese, President Nixon told the American people that all U.S. POWs are now free.

"For the first time in 12 years, we can observe Armed Forces Day with all of our fighting forces home from Vietnam and all of our courageous prisoners of war set free and here back home in America," said Nixon in a speech on May 19, 1973. Did he really believe that?

What about Kissinger?

"Once Kissinger had concluded his discussions and negotiations in 1973, it was a dead issue," concluded Larry Stark, a civilian employee of the U.S. Navy in Vietnam who was taken prisoner by the North Vietnamese. He was a POW from 1968 to 1973.

If the hunt for America's POW/MIAs failed because of politics, can a grassroots effort help resolve the issue?

"Yes," says Captain McDainel, "if the American people push hard for action. Politicians only react, they don't act."

Gen. Tighe blames the American people for allowing the U.S. government to abandon POW/MIAs in Southeast Asia.

At a congressional hearing on POW/MIAs in 1981, Tighe, then director of the DIA, testified that there were still likely to be American POWs in Southeast Asia. He wonders why the American people didn't jump on the issue.

"It's up to them to decide whether this is an issue or not," Tighe says. But the American people can only do so much. The POW/MIA issue is a political football.

"It appears that the entire issue is being manipulated by unscrupulous people in the government, or associated with the government," DIA's POW/MIA Chief Peck stated when he quit his job. "Some are using the issue for personal or political advantage and others use it as a forum to perform and feel important, or worse."

"The sad fact, however, is that the issue is being controlled and a cover-up may be in progress. The entire charade does not appear to be an honest effort, and may never have been," Peck says.

DoD intelligence reports from the Vietnam War, post-war live-sightings, reports and photographs that appear to be of MIAs, have led many people to believe that the United States abandoned some of its servicemen in Southeast Asia. Tighe, Peck and Mooney are among those who believe that.

Since the end of the war in 1973, DoD has compiled about 1,500 first-hand live-sighting reports and 5,000 second and third-hand reports. According to the Pentagon's *1991 POW/MIA Fact Book*, only about 100 of these are considered "believable."

Nevertheless, the thousands of boat people who fled Vietnam came to the United States with information on American POWs. Peck said that the government expends more effort discrediting sources than it does checking out their information.

Despite the Pentagon's dismissal of most refugee stories, many of them reveal compelling, detailed information about U.S. POWs. And many reports corroborate previous sightings.

For example, DoD reports chronicled consistent accounts of U.S. POWs in a prison near the town of Bat Bat, 60 miles from Hanoi, after the war. They cite a high-ranking North Vietnamese policeman who claimed he saw several U.S. POWs inside the camp while he repaired the fence. They also cited a North Vietnamese doctor who said he provided medical treatment for U.S. pilots. Both accounts cover a specific area and were obtained independently.

Another example: A Feburary 23, 1979, Joint Casualty Resolution Center (JCRC) memo reports that a refugee interviewed on Feb. 14, 1979, said she saw Caucasians working on a road in Vietnam's Song Be Province.

The JCRC, established by the Joint Chiefs of Staff in 1983, is responsible for pursuing an accounting of American POW/MIAs in Southeast Asia.

According to the memo, the Caucasians told the refugee, "There are 30 Americans kept here. We all need food. If you bring food for us, the American government will reward you."

Dead or alive, it isn't easy to get information on American POW/MIAs in Southeast Asia. Most of it is classified. In fact, much of this data is so classified that no one can act on it.

The overall U.S. government policy on POW/MIAs is coordinated through the POW/MIA Inter-Agency Group (IAG), an umbrella organization of government agencies that includes the DoD, the White House JSC staff, the State Department, the Joint Chiefs of Staff (JCS), the DIA and the National League of POW/MIA Families.

Some agencies, like the DIA, just collect information and classify it as it comes in. Others, like DoD, are empowered to act on it, if they know about it.

"From the beginning of the (Vietnam) war to about mid-1970, there was a vast amount of information that was suppressed, which contained a lot of detail about POWs," says Mooney.

"Several thousand intercepts were never properly processed and sent anywhere, except they remained right at the agency level between 1965 and 1970," he told *The American Legion* magazine.

"There's a black hole between 1965 and 1970, where none of the data went forward," Mooney says.

"Since POW/MIA information was so highly classified, it did not get to the right people," Mooney says. "Consequently, people died. The data should have gone right to the tactical commanders, the fighter wing commanders, the route infantry commanders, where it could have been acted on immediately."

Mooney says that the information never reached the people who could take action. Most of the POW/MIA intelligence was quickly classified and filed by the DIA.

The DIA director reports directly to the Secretary of Defense and Chairman of the Joint Chiefs of Staff. Either official can authorize a POW/MIA search, but the DIA cannot act on the intelligence it receives.

"The DIA is not an action-oriented agency," General Tighe confirms. He says that the DIA is primarily a collector of intelligence—classifying it, analyzing it and passing it on to other agencies.

So who can act on POW/MIA intelligence generated by the DIA?

"Whomever the Joint Chiefs of Staff directs to do so, " Tighe says. "They can ask any of the services to do it. They can ask all kinds of organizations to do what they want done. But (they should be) organizations that have military action-oriented people."

It's a question of honor. The Cold War may be over, but highly classified U.S. government files still hold the last secrets of the Vietnam War, particularly the fate of POW/MIAs.

According to the U.S. Information Security Oversight Office (ISOO), the U. S. government has 7 million classified documents. And only 3 percent of these will ever be released to the public. If World War I troop movements are still classified—and they are—why would the U.S. government ever release its politically sensitive POW/MIA intelligence?

"What we're trying to do is solve something that's akin to a 20-year-old crime," says General Vessey.

But all the clues are classified.

"It's time for the U.S. government to declassify its information on American POW/MIAs," says DiFrancesco. "There is no earthly reason why a matter which has been assigned 'the highest national priority' should remain buried in the bowels of our government while more than 2,000 American families are suffering."

The families of 2,267 Americans have something in common: a missing member. And in the shadow of America's longest and most unpopular war—Vietnam—they go through life not knowing what happened to their sons, husbands, fathers and brothers.

Has the U.S. abandoned POWs in Southeast Asia?

Today, the fate of America's "missing" hangs on one issue: the road map, the plan to re-establish relations with Vietnam.

To help rebuild Vietnam's economy with financial aid, trade and diplomatic relations, some say, is the best way to get information on our POW/MIAs.

To others, the road map is a death sentence for America's missing men.

According to DiFrancesco, "To give Vietnam what it wants now, without a full accounting, would seal the last secrets of the Vietnam War forever."

The Department of Defense POW/MIA Newsletter of March 1992, reported that ". . . on November 5, 1991, Secretary of Defense Dick Cheney became the first Secretary of Defense to testify before Congress on the POW/MIA issue." Secretary Cheney stated:

"I can think of no subject that stirs more emotion or generates more frustration and controversy than the subject of prisoners of war and missing in action, especially those lost during our operations in Southeast Asia.

"The fact that there were thousands unaccounted for in previous wars does not make it any easier to accept the fact that 18 years after active U.S. participation in the Vietnam War ended, we still do not have a full accounting of all those lost in combat.

"When we defeated Iraqi forces in the gulf in February 1991, we were able to account for all our people, even those lost behind enemy lines. That achievement is one of the legacies of our concern for our missing . . . ."

Secretary Cheney's testimony was comprehensive and covered all aspects of the POW/MIA issue. From on-going negotiations with the governments of Indochina, to current recovery operations in Southeast Asia, live-sighting investigations and the creation of a military organization in the United States Pacific Command to expand U.S. POW/MIA operation in Southeast Asia commensurate with cooperation provided by the government of Indochina.

The National League of Families of American Prisoners and Missing in Southeast Asia is a staunch advocate of responsible, factual public awareness and education on the POW/MIA issue. It has been through this process that increased pressure has involved on both the U.S. and Southeast Asian government to seriously address the questions which still remain.

According to Mary C. Backley, Director of Operations and Public Relations for the National League of Families of American Prisoners and Missing in Southeast Asia, ". . . the League originated on the west coast in the late 1960s. The wife of a ranking POW, believing that the U.S. government's policy of keeping a low profile on the POW/MIA issue and encouraging the families to refrain from publicly discussing the problem was unjustified, initiated a loosely-organized movement which eventually developed into the National League of Families."

Membership is comprised solely of the wives, children, parents and other close relatives of Americans who were or are listed as POW, MIA, KIA and BNR (body not recovered) in Southeast Asia, and returned Vietnam POWs.

The League's sole purpose, as published in its newsletter, is to obtain the release of all prisoners, the fullest possible accounting for the missing and the repatriation of all recoverable remains of those who died serving our nation in Southeast Asia. It is a non-profit, non-partisan organization financed through contributions from the families, concerned citizens and organizations. The membership now stands at over 3,800.

The position stated is that Americans are being held against their will in Southeast Asia and has been since incorporation, as stated publicly on numerous occasions. As we are all aware, the families have waited far too long to obtain answers on their missing loved ones—alive or dead; however, it is important to note that the League has been through a great deal (five administrations) and recognizes the difference between current seriousness on the part of the U.S. government versus past apathy and indifference from previous administrations. For years, the families fought for our own government's attention. This was met with inaccurate information, blatant falsehoods and inaction until 1982.

The newsletter continues: President Reagan came into office with an established commitment to pursue resolution of the POW/MIA issue as a matter of highest national priority and concern. This is also a commitment of the Bush administration and, apparently, the current administration based on statements conveyed by President Clinton during his campaign.

Intelligence assets, resources and priorities were raised to a level which should have been pursued in earlier years, but were not. Increased intelligence collection has brought over 1,600 first-hand live-sighting reports of individuals the sources believe to be American prisoners in various stages of control, from actual captivity to moving freely in a given area.

According to the League's newsletter, while the past several years of priority efforts (1982–present) have thus far produced no living Americans, over 240 families have received answers through government-to-government efforts (no Americans have been accounted for through private efforts.)

Again, the League continues to press for the return of live Americans. The fullest possible accounting is crucial to achieving answers for the families and directly impacts the live-prisoner issue. The two tracks must be pursued simultaneously.

In addition, the League is directly responsible for the change in U.S. government policy on the POW/MIA issue, particularly concerning living prisoners of war.

The POW/MIA issue is a bi-partisan issue and receives strong support across the board in Congress.

In a June 11, 1992 letter to Secretary Cheney, the League's Executive Director Ann Mills Griffiths said:

"As a result of the last League board of directors meeting and on their behalf, I am writing to express concern over the lack of results from the Vietnamese in terms of accounting for missing Americans.

"This is especially relevant when compared with the increased level of joint field activities in Vietnam. The League recognizes and appreciates the commitment of assets and resources; however, I'm confident that you agree with us that activity is not a substitute for results.

"Despite this, a pro-active media effort has succeeded in bringing positive exposure to the expanded U.S. field effort, but not to the fact that final answers are minimal, i.e. only three Americans were accounted for as a result of U.S./SRV joint cooperation during 1991.

"In the absence of unilateral SRV remains repatriations and adequate U.S. access to Vietnam's wartime records, including those which pertain to U.S. losses in Laos (over 80% of 522) and Cambodia (90% of 83), we view U.S. policy as being poorly served by heaping unwarranted praise on the Vietnamese.

"Public misperception can only be advantageous to the government of Vietnam and those who advocate lifting the economic embargo despite the lack of more serious Vietnamese cooperation to resolve the issue."

Secretary Cheney responded:

"While I applaud Vietnam's willingness to engage in increased levels of activity, they are well aware that the only way to move forward with normalization is via the policy embedded in the 'road map' which is explicit in terms of required results.

"I believe the key to all of this is in effective planning and implementation of constructive activity, while insisting that the Vietnamese be forthcoming with information which will enhance results.

"Until I am satisfied with the results in Vietnam, I will continue to move cautiously down the road map to normalization."

According to the League's newsletter of January 1993, 2,261 Americans are still missing as a result of the Vietnam War. A breakdown by country of loss follows: Vietnam 1,644 (North–602; South–1,052); Laos–519; Cambodia–80; Chinese territorial water–8. Over 80% of Laos and 90% of Cambodia losses occurred in areas controlled by Vietnamese forces during the war.

At the forefront of negotiations and intelligence efforts since 1982 is resolving the live-prisoner issue. The League's position is that Americans are known to have been left behind in captivity in Vietnam, Laos and Cambodia. In the absence of evidence to the contrary, it can only be assumed that these Americans remain alive in captivity today.

The League states its position on POW/MIAs as the following: "As a matter of policy, the USG operates under the assumption that U.S. POWs could still be held, a position recently affirmed by the Senate Select Committee on POW/MIA Affairs."

Recognizing the importance of POW/MIA-related criteria in the U.S. "road map" to improved relations with Vietnam, the League supports such an approach, providing significant leverage is not lost, as would be by taking International Monetary Fund-related steps, until Vietnam acts unilaterally and rapidly to resolve last-known alive cases and repatriate remains readily available.

Robert D. Norris, a Tulsa Attorney and military historian, says:

"The Tet Offensive of January and February of 1968 was the pivotal event of the Vietnam War. What was in reality a bloody defeat for the Viet Cong and North Vietnamese Army, was turned into a propaganda victory by the misreporting of the elite American media, which broke the will of Lyndon Johnson and exhausted the patience of the American public. The year that followed saw the bloodiest fighting in the war.

"Ironically, because the battles of Tet were inconclusive, they condemned the Americans and South Vietnamese to five more years of war. The American government was trapped in a morass which it had neither the courage to quit nor the will to win.

"The result was a bloody stalemate. Both sides tried to exhaust the other in a series of pitched, bloody, yet indecisive battles.

"In the stalemate, American morale plummeted; nobody could argue that the fighting was for anything tangible. The North Vietnamese Army took horrific losses as the intransigent leadership in Hanoi (which understood the American politicians better than they understood themselves) flung hordes of ground troops into the meat-grinder of

American firepower, trading lives for time and the inevitable loss of American patience.

"Ironically, while the American public had no stomach for a stalemate, public opinion polls showed that they would have supported the government had it decisively moved to win the war through the application of overwhelming force and knock-out blows to the enemy. Washington continued to vacillate, with disastrous consequences.

"Some of the grimmest days in American military history, in which many Americans were killed or captured, was sobering and cautionary in light of the fact that while the military learned the lessons of Vietnam, many of our current leaders have not."

This is just one of the hundreds of important battles where Americans were killed and/or captured. These same POW/MIAs are the focal point of the issue today.

One might wonder, how on earth can relations with Vietnam, Laos and Cambodia be normal? Consider this . . .

Vietnam's Wish List	USA's Wish List
Mobile Oil	Billy Jack Cartwright, USN
NBC/CBS/ABC	Winfield W. Sisson, USMC
McDonalds	Humberto Acosta-Rosario, USA
Shell	Victor Joe Apodaca, Jr. USAF
IBM	Roy F. Townley
Citibanc	Jack C. Ritticher, USCG
Hilton Hotels	Donald G. Carr, USA
General Motors	Anthony Giannangeli, USAF
Int'l Monetary Funds . . .	Wayne Bibbs, USA
	James Kelly Patterson, USN
	Anthony C. Shine, USAF
	Michael John Shea, USMC
	and hundreds more. . . .

Joel H. Cook served in Vietnam from January 1970 to March 1971. Serving "in Country," Cook was exposed to Agent Orange, a chemical used by the United States military as a defoliant during the war.

Earlier, the man who has worked for the return of the many in Vietnam, brought a part of that place home with him, in the form of Soft Tissue Sarcomas. Cook has a long and large battle ahead of him, filled with radiation treatments and surgery. Taking a break from stressing the importance of POW/MIAs, Cook now stresses to veterans that they should be administered an Agent Orange test.

"I thought I was invincible," said Cook. "If it can hit me, it can hit others. It's a little late for me, but not for them."

In a recent article in the *Walkill Valley Times*, reporter Kathleen Aris visited with Joel as he reflected over the past 15 years of his life. Between working a full-time job and raising two children with his wife, Linda, Cook took a stand and dedicated himself to fighting for the 2,267 American soldiers listed as missing in action or as prisoners of war in Vietnam.

His dream of bringing one of those soldiers home ended recently, when he retired as head of the National Human Rights Committee for POW/MIAs and asked that the organization be disbanded.

The Executive Board of the National Human Rights Committee for POW/MIAs voted unanimously to disband, at Cook's request. (Unable to keep up with the demanding schedule of spreading public awareness and speaking engagements because of his ill health, Cook asked the committee to end its efforts and liquidate the remainder of the committee's fundraising. The committee of 3,200 completely disbanded.)

The National Human Rights Committee for POW/MIAs was formed on July 7, 1977, with Cook's attentions focusing on a local organization in Walden, New York, that would make the public aware of those missing in action or held as prisoners of war. More than just a veterans group, the committee was more of a public awareness organization reminding the public, "If you don't care, who will?"

Information learned through Cook's persistence and diligence has been turned over to the federal government and the National League of Families and has led to a national network of citizens spreading the words, "Lest We Forget" through bumper stickers and flags.

Cook's interest in Americans still in Vietnam was sparked by the lack of support shown by citizens as he attended a rally in Washington, D.C. (Less than 50 people attended the rally to show their concern for American military in Vietnam. Cook's outrage by the poor attendance at the rally led to a 15-year fight for POW/MIAs' rights and lives.)

"We're not going to let it die," Cook said to the person he attended the rally with—the mother of a missing soldier. "I'm going to do something— even if it's small."

After a small amount of publicity, the first meeting was held, with more than 50 people attending. They came from all over the area, all over New York state, and some from as far as Pennsylvania, with one purpose in mind. Cook was on his way in forming a local group to spread the word about POW/MIAs. People attending the meeting weren't happy that it was just going to be a local effort. They wanted something more, a national work force.

"At first I thought I would bite off more than I could chew, but I figured we might as well go all the way," Cook says. "We wanted to do it in a professional way, and we did it."

After the first materials citing the group's purpose were circulated all over the country, responses came pouring in. "People couldn't believe Americans were still over there," Cook says. Politicians and journalists, seeking information and wishing to assist in the fight, began calling and writing to Cook and the committee.

"We were anti-government when we first started, right up to when Reagan was elected because the government was covering up the issue," Cook says. "We pushed for Carter to be elected since we were discouraged with the Republicans. When he came into office, Carter just about killed the whole issue, saying there was no proof there were any Americans there."

Cook says, "Reagan worked with POWs who came home in 1973, and our hopes were up. He met with families and said how embarrassed he was about past administrations and how the issue was handled. He promised it would be one of his top priorities, and while he didn't get anyone home, he did find out where people were. Bush followed in Reagan's footsteps."

In his tenure as president of the committee, Cook saw that public awareness was spread regarding the issue, and said people know what POW/MIA means. The POW/MIA flag flies throughout the country and in Canada, and is even displayed in the Capital rotunda in Washington, D.C.

Rallies of support have been held, and Cook believes work to bring more information out of Vietnam regarding POW/MIAs is surfacing at a faster pace now. The federal government currently has a temporary office in Vietnam, something that wasn't always there that is keeping relations and work with that country's officials moving forward. The work of the committee and organizations like it have aided in the fight to bring Americans home.

"Citizens now know we still have people unaccounted for," Cook says. "Because of our work and other organizations' efforts, everyone who went to Desert Storm has been accounted for. The government is not covering this up. What people don't understand is the reports that come in are five to six years old, and there are more coming in, some as young as a month, but no one sees them. This is the stuff we're up against."

While he said he's not sorry about any of his actions over the past 15 years, Cook does believe more time should have been given to his wife and their two children, Steven and Rachel.

Cook does have one regret though. Tearfully, he wished he could have seen one come out.

"If it's only one, we owe it to him or her to get them back alive," he said. "And if not, we owe it to their families to get their remains so that they know."

The VFW Commander-in-Chief, John M. Carney said, "For more than a quarter century, the VFW has been in the vanguard of the fight for the veterans of Vietnam. That battle has been waged on several fronts, ranging from passage of legislation, support for GIs during the war, contributions to the Vietnam Veterans Memorial and continuing efforts to resolve the fate of the war's missing in action."

Contrary to popular belief, Vietnam veterans were not shunned by all sectors of society. They were American fighting men. They answered the call of their country.

To obtain firsthand information on how the search for GIs missing from the Vietnam War was going, VFW's Junior Vice Commander-in-Chief, Allen "Gunner" Kent, and VFW Washington Office Executive Director, Larry Rivers, recently visited Southeast Asia. Here is an account of their trip:

The countries they visited in Southeast Asia were Thailand, Vietnam and Laos. Their November trip was scheduled to coincide with the visit made by members of the Senate Select Committee on POW/MIA Affairs. This gave them the opportunity to observe the meetings between the U.S. senators and Vietnamese officials.

They reported that the Americans assigned to the duty of searching for traces of GIs unaccounted for from the war worked tirelessly under the most unpleasant circumstances. The public must know of their sacrifices and commitment. They are truly heroes.

The resolution of the POW/MIA issue really became a national priority with the appointment of Vessey as special emissary to Vietnam in 1987. He revitalized and energized government efforts and for that we are in his debt.

The Joint Task Force-Full Accounting (JTF-FA) is successor to the Joint Casualty Resolution Center. It was formed in February 1992, and comprises four detachments based in Bangkok, Hanoi, Vientiane and Phnom Penh.

A unit called Stoney Beach, located in the U.S. Embassy in Bangkok, is tasked with the mission of collecting intelligence with full strength of 25 personnel.

The function of the Detachment 2 in Hanoi is to perform historical research, investigate live-sighting reports, conduct excavations and participate in technical meetings, among other duties.

Joint Field Activity (JFA) is actual field investigations. They last about 30 days. Over 20 have been conducted in Vietnam to date with varying degrees of success. Others have taken place in Laos and Cambodia.

On-scene observers rate the level of cooperation of the Vietnamese as adequate. All agree that more can be done, but the cumbersome Communist bureaucracy is a major impediment to progress.

In Hanoi, the regime there insists that cooperation on the POW/MIA issue would be "enhanced" by the establishment of diplomatic relations. Clearly, this is the end result it desires—normalization of political and economic ties.

When questioned about living Americans, the director of the Vietnam Office For Seeking Missing Persons says there is simply not a shred of credible evidence to suggest Americans are being held.

According to the Senate Select Committee, 44 credible live-sightings exist; of which 29 have been investigated in Vietnam.

Vietnam is giving remains recovery and repatriation little attention until all the 135 discrepancy cases have been resolved. (Ninety-six are near settlement.) Holding back on this issue, in Vietnam's estimation, is the quickest road to normalization of relations. Still, the Vietnamese deny warehousing or otherwise holding remains.

The situation in Laos is that the military there does not trust the U.S. motives. Therefore, investigations are limited by that government.

There are some significant developments on the horizon. Access to museums and other archives could yield some good leads. The fact that the Vietnamese government pledges to continue working with us is significant. We will also soon have detachments in Da Nang and Ho Chi Minh City.

It was reported that there is a North Vietnamese/Viet Cong veterans group forming in Vietnam. We should monitor the progress of this group which might help in solving the POW/MIA issue.

Wondering if it is realistic to expect a full accounting of all lost GIs, we must accept the fact that some cases will never be fully resolved. That's just a hard truth. Due to time, lack of witnesses, rugged terrain and climatic conditions—as was the case with WWII and Korea—the remains of many MIAs are impossible to find.

One American is still classified as a POW. U.S. Air Force Col. Charles E. Shelton was shot down over Laos on April 29, 1965, and is kept in this status as a symbolic gesture of the U.S. government's commitment to continue the search.

We must revise the guidelines and devise a realistic mechanism that allows, when appropriate, for cases to be resolved without actually finding a live American or his remains.

In regard to normalizing relations with Vietnam, VFW resolutions call for the fullest cooperation in resolving the POW/MIA issue prior to even considering establishment of diplomatic relations and/or economic aid.

What constitutes full cooperation is verification that the Vietnamese are indeed allowing full and unfettered access to archival materials and unrestricted travel in the countryside to search for remains for as long as necessary.

Findings of the Senate Select Committee on POW/MIA Affairs, released in a report on January 13, 1993, after a $2 million and 15-month investigation, produced some expected conclusions.

The unanimous report, despite last minute wrangling, is the most comprehensive effort ever undertaken to resolve the fate of America's 2,267 still unaccounted for GIs from the Vietnam War.

The 585-page document was completed after making several trips to Indochina, reviewing 1 million pages of previously classified documents, holding 23 public hearings and interviewing nearly 200 witnesses under oath.

The committee determined:

- No "specific" evidence exists that any American POWs were knowingly left behind after the war.

- No compelling proof exists that U.S. POWs are still alive in Indochina.

- Con-artists have exploited the POW/MIA situation and should be prosecuted for fraud.

- Successive administrations did not deal forthrightly with POW/MIA families.

- Some U.S. POWs may have survived in Laos after the Paris Peace Accords, but this issue was "shunted aside and discounted by government and population alike."

- The Pentagon's effort was sometimes flawed.

- Twenty years of intransigence by Hanoi has kept the issue alive among the public.

The report concluded: "The bottom line is that there remain only a few cases where we know an unreturned POW was alive in captivity and we do not have evidence that the individual also died in captivity."

New Hampshire Senator Robert C. Smith and Iowa Senator Charles E. Grassley filed exceptions to some of the conclusions about live-sightings.

General William C. Westmoreland outlined his views on Vietnam and its aftermath. Retired since 1972, Gen. Westmoreland was Commander of U.S. forces in Vietnam from 1964 through June 1968. During World War II, he served with the 9th Infantry Division in Tunisia, Sicily, France, Belgium and Germany. During the war in Korea, he commanded the 187th Regimental Combat Team.

General Westmoreland said:

"The Paris Peace Accords were not worth the paper they were written on. The agreement was not concluded in good faith by the Vietnamese. Henry Kissinger and then-President Richard Nixon went for it because it was the easier route out of Vietnam.

"If the Vietnam War was winnable at a reasonable price in American lives is a very complex question. We certainly had the military power to win it, but if we had exercised that power, which we were capable of doing, there was a better than 50-50 chance that the Chinese would have come to the battlefield. If the Chinese had come to the battlefield, that would not necessarily mean that we would have lost the war, but it would have meant a tremendous cost in lives and resources.

"Communist propaganda was able to transform the Tet Offensive—which was a devastating military debacle for the Communists—into a brilliant victory for Hanoi. Tet was a massive defeat for North Vietnam. However, the media overreacted to the extent of damage inflicted by the enemy.

"I briefed them and explained what actually occurred, but they never admitted or corrected their misjudgement. Television was a major factor in that, as in much of the coverage of the war.

"There were few reporters who had the credibility with the military and whom we believed gave the military a fair break, but there were none of the stature and ability of Ernie Pyle.

"Comparing the fighting abilities, dedication and morale with those of World War II and Korea, our troops in Vietnam were excellent. I have nothing but pride in the way they fought in spite of the fact that they did not have enthusiastic support here at home, as our troops had in World War II and, to an extent, in Korea.

"One may wonder if the Americans who served in Vietnam were vindicated by the war's ultimate outcome. The troops who served there did what the country asked them to do and did it admirably under the most difficult circumstances that our country ever asked our soldiers to tolerate.

"Not only the climate, but the nature of the enemy and also the fact that they didn't have a world of support from the people at home affected the outcome.

In light of what transpired in Vietnam, Cambodia and Laos in the last 20 years, I have no doubts in the least, about the rightness of U.S. intentions in Vietnam. There was a strong, positive result of our commitment there, in that we stopped the pressure of communism toward Southeast Asia.

"In the early days of Ho Chi Minh, a campaign was designed with the support of Communist China, to spread communism down to the Malacca Straits through the Asian countries.

"The thrust of communism was blocked by our commitment. Many do not appreciate that natural resource-wise, Southeast Asia is probably the wealthiest part of the world. In addition, that area controls the very few sea lanes from Asia to the Indian Ocean.

"It is an absolute fact that America's stance in Southeast Asia bought time for other Asian nations to develop economically and evolve politically.

"At least in part, because of America's persistence in Indochina, the Free World won a wider victory (i.e., the collapse of European communism). It had an impact, there's no question about that. Our NATO forces facing the Soviet Communists played a very important strategic role on behalf of our country and on behalf of the free world. Also, our stand in Vietnam manifested that same objective.

"We've heard much about the so-called lessons of Vietnam. Considering the U.S.'s involvement in Beirut (1983), the situation in Iraq and calls for 'limited' U.S. military intervention in the former Yugoslavia, this nation's leadership should have learned that military power has to be used for political purposes and ideological purposes from time to time.

"The world is now, basically, safe for democracy primarily because of the United States military. Without the U.S. military, we would have an entirely different world today.

"I wouldn't say the President or the Secretary of Defense, who did not serve during wartime, has the moral authority; he has the moral responsibility to protect the United States' interests. I believe Mr. Clinton, although he did not ever serve in uniform and his political orientation during certain stages of our international activities was not compatible with many of us at that time, now has the 'monkey on his back.'

"He is the Commander-in-Chief and shoulders the American interest to which he has to give his primary attention. As Commander-in-Chief, I believe he will act responsibly in the national interest.

"I think we are moving in the direction of establishing full diplomatic relations with Vietnam. We've opened the door to trade relations now, as I understand it. The next step, I think, will be diplomatic relations which we have not yet done and which I would hesitate to support until we have, among other things, a commitment from Hanoi on the POW/MIA issue, and when we are convinced they are doing everything they can to come clean on that issue.

"I do not think the United States should pay war reparations (i.e., economic aid) to Hanoi. Recognizing the regime in Hanoi—the same one that violated every precept of the Paris Peace Accords—would vindicate the position of the anti-war movement. I would hesitate to establish diplomatic relations with them until they change their form of government. I don't believe that we can trust a Communist government.

"The question has been asked—have Vietnam veterans finally been accorded genuine respect by society or is lip service being paid Vietnam vets to assuage a national guilt complex? I think there is an appreciation of the role of the Vietnam veteran that didn't exist five years ago and certainly didn't exist 10 or 20 years ago. That's also reflected in the attitude of the Vietnam veterans themselves.They knew they did what this country asked them to do and nobody could have done it better.

"As far as how Vietnam veterans will be treated in American history books, I think they will be treated fairly, positively and with admiration.

I have no doubt about that."

Mack M. Brooks, Lt. Col. U.S. Army Chief of POW/MIA Affairs says, "These questions are very complex and contentious. In large part, they were the subject of a year-long inquiry by the Senate Select Committee on POW/MIA Affairs in 1992 and earlier hearings by House of Representatives Committee on Veterans Affairs (1986) and Committee on Foreign Affairs (1988).

These sources should be able to supply the fullest possible assessment of what transpired concerning the Vietnam era regarding POW/MIAs."

Washington-based Cliff Kincaid, who writes for *Human Events* and other publications, says that President Clinton is being flooded with letters asking him to keep his word that there will be no diplomatic recognition of Hanoi and no lifting of the trade embargo until there is the fullest possible accounting of the POW/MIA issue.

The Senate Select Committee on POW/MIA Affairs spent more than a year on the issue, ambiguously concluding that some Americans may have been left behind after Vietnam.

Its final report was marred by the revelation that Henry Kissinger's lawyer was allowed to review and alter an early draft.

President Clinton is said to feel no pressure to improve relations with Vietnam while there are unanswered questions about missing Americans. Some activists want Clinton to appoint Ross Perot to head another commission to resolve the issue.

Part 2

How long shall I have perplexity in my mind,
and grief in my heart, day after day?
How long shall my enemy triumph over me?

Psalms 13:2

The Black Wall

He lost his life in '66
It seems so long ago,
You'd think I'd have forgotten by now
But you see, it is not so.
We all were good Americans,
Answering our country's call,
We went to war, sure that we were right,
Oh, we stood so proud and tall.
We were the 'Nam Quixotes
Tilting at those Asian mills,
We gave our all, the best we had.
It was kill or else be killed.
And when it ended we came home.
To scorn and taunts and hate.
Having lost our youth and closest friends.
Unsure as to our fate.
But in my dreams I'm still in 'Nam.
His face is sharp and clear.
And we still laugh and reminisce
Of home and those held dear.
For me, my friend can never die.
There just can be no way.
He's with me in my heart of hearts.
Every minute of each day.
For every name on that black wall.
I'm sure there's more like me.
To whom the man behind the name
Is a cherished memory.

Carl J. Decker
Written in memory of Capt. James P. Williams
USMC. KIA. Tam Quan. Republic of Vietnam. 3/66.

Did We Leave
POW/MIAs Behind?

There are undoubtly many reasons behind the reluctance of officials to look seriously at the allegations of those most directly involved in the POW/MIA issue.

But, rather than make sweeping generalizations, let us take a look at what some of the most renowned, respected and qualified Americans have to say on the subject. Each were asked the following five questions:

1. Did we knowingly leave prisoners in Southeast Asia when our forces left?
2. Are some of these prisoners still alive?
3. What should our government have done at the time?
4. What should our government do now?
5. How have your thoughts about these questions changed over the past 20 years?

The quotations that follow are as diverse as the personalities who authored them. They illustrate, if nothing else, the great range and depth of men's thinking on the near 20-year enigma of "POW/MIAs—AMERICA'S MISSING MEN."

Robinson "Robbie" Risner:
- Brig. Gen. USAF (Ret.).
- Thirty-three years Service. More than 100 combat missions in Korea.
- He was shot down twice, becoming America's 20th Jet ace by shooting down eight Soviet-made fighters.
- He set the transatlantic speed record during a 30th anniversary commemoration of Charles Linberg's solo flight.
- During the Vietnam War, he was shot down twice over North Vietnam. The second time he was captured and held in the "Hanoi Hilton" and "Heartbreak Hotel" for seven and a half years.
- Author: *The Passing Of The Night*, dedicated to the youth of America, describing his Air Force experiences, concentration on the time spent as POW.
- He was the first living recipient of the Air Force's highest award, the Air Force Cross (twice). Sixty-five Awards and Decorations including, the Distinguished Service Medal, three Distinguished Flying Crosses, the Bronze Star with V for Valor, two Silver Stars, eight Air Medals and three Purple Hearts.

- Enshrined in both the Oklahoma Hall of Fame and Space Museum.
- He received the Oklahoma Cross of Valor Medal and Honorary Doctor-of-Law Degree from Oklahoma Christian College.
- Organized and served as the Executive Director of the "Texan's War on Drugs" for four years and was appointed by President Ronald Reagan as a United States Representative to the 40th Session of the United States General Assembly.

"Did our government knowingly leave American POWs in Southeast Asia when we left in 1973? Yes! As a member of an oversight committee on POW/MIA Affairs, I spent two weeks in the basement of the DIA reviewing hundreds of live-sighting reports.

"In addition to convincing evidence, I figured that 41 percent of the American Airmen shot down over North Vietnam and not rescued, survived and were repatriated. I applied the same percentage figure to the 567 Airmen shot down over Laos and arrived at a figure of 232 men that became POW/MIAs in Laos. With the exception of three men who were captured by North Vietnamese regulars or turned over to them, not one POW was ever repatriated from Laos.

"Judging from personal knowledge of the survival capabilities of American POWs, plus the live-sightings in later years, I feel that some of the American POW/MIAs are still alive in Southeast Asia.

"At the time the peace agreements were being drawn up, the PL (Pathet Lao) government should have been brought into the negotiations. As far as I know, this was never done.

"Our government should start immediately to negotiate with the Pathet Lao, using whatever means necessary to free those American fighting men.

"For several years after I was repatriated (Feburary 12, 1973), our government emphasized that **all** American POW/MIAs held in Southeast Asia had been brought home—and I believed them.

"I know now, that they were not telling the truth. Even Yeltsin of Russia, plus the KGB General who defected to America, say that American POW/MIAs were sent to the USSR, plus more were still being held in Vietnam years after the war was over."

John McCain:
- United States Senator.
- Member of the Senate Select Committee on POW/MIA Affairs.

"As a member of the Senate Select Committee on POW/MIA Affairs, I had the opportunity to review more information on our missing servicemen than at any other time in my career. If my views on this matter have changed at all over the last 20 years, they have come to reflect a more studied perspective.

"Throughout the deliberations of the Senate Select Committee, I saw no evidence that American servicemen were left behind in Southeast Asia, knowingly or otherwise.

"As evidenced by former Secretary of State Henry Kissinger's testimony, the options that were open to American policy makers at the time were very limited. But, precipitous and unwise action in Congress severely weakened the Nixon administration's negotiation position at the Paris peace talks. Under the circumstances, I believe the administration did all it could.

"We must continue to make the fullest possible accounting of our servicemen a condition to normalization of relations with Vietnam.

"Assistant Secretary Solomon's 'road map' to normalization remains our most reliable guide to forging a new relationship with our old adversary. Recent cooperation on the POW/MIA issue is encouraging, but we must continue to press for a fuller accounting."

Dwight Perry:
- Vietnam Veteran 1967-1970.
- Second 28th Infantry, 1st Infantry Division, Delta Company.
- Combat Infantryman's Badge, Commendation for Heroism, two Purple Hearts, two Bronze Stars, Air Medal, Expert Rifleman, M-16, M-14, 45 Cal. Disabled Vietnam Veteran.

"So many thoughts have crossed my mind over the years regarding my personal experiences while in Vietnam. I have also tried to do quite a bit of investigating regarding our POW/MIA issue.

"I have personally felt a tremendous load of guilt as though I had personally let my fellow soldiers down, as a result of abandoning them when we pulled out. This guilt has been but another load to carry along with all the other problems as a result of experiencing Vietnam.

"Yes, I do believe we 'the U.S. government' knowingly left prisoners at the time of pull out. While I do believe there are or was, those who may have stayed as a result of their own free will, I do not believe there are any prisoners who might still be alive. That environment is just too hostile to endure such a treatment for so long.

"I think this subject is just another example of this fine, upstanding government's ineptness, and downright criminal activity, both then and now, and in between. My faith in this government and people we went to war for has been stomped on, ridiculed, and ostracized these many years.

"For so many years, I believed in what our government officials said and what we were taught as youngsters growing up. Now, I believe that if you can hear a politician's voice, he's lying.

"When this country can elect a draft dodger, wife cheater, and a liar to boot for President, then I've lost all my respect for what we did in Vietnam. It's all a mockery."

Barry R. McCaffrey:
- Lt. General, U.S. Army.
- Assistant to Colin Powell, Joint Chief of Staff, Washington, D.C.

"We can never conclusively rule out that some of our servicemen were kept at the end of World War II, Korea or Vietnam. The overwhelming majority of our MIA were, without doubt, killed-in-action and lie in a lost soldier's grave on some foreign battlefield. Others may have been executed by brutal captors or died of maltreatment.

"A combination of political and human dynamics has kept the issue of the Vietnam MIAs painfully alive over the long years since the end of the war. The issue has been shamelessly exploited by some for political or financial gain.

"Each revelation subjects the families to new uncertainty. The lingering ideological warfare of the Vietnam experience creates conspiracy theories which hold successive U.S. adminstrations to be part of a continuing deception.

"The North Vietnamese never have given us an adequate accounting of the POW/MIAs. However, we now have a good mechanism in place in Hanoi to resolve the list of missing name-by-name.

"Bandits and con-artists in Southeast Asia continue to feed bits of hope to desperate families. However, in my judgement, there is no credible evidence that U.S. POWs are held in post-war Vietnam. This does not argue that it could not have happened, only that no intelligence withstands close scrutiny.

"In my estimation, no U.S. prisoners remain in captivity from World War II, Korea or Vietnam. Those of us in uniform would argue loudly and publicly for decisive political and military action to gain the release of any possible POWs.

"There will be one last roll call. I am sure of that. On that day we shall again all stand together in the ranks of our regiments and learn how each of our MIA met his fate. We don't know the pain of death. We certainly remember the honor of their lives."

Leon E. Briggs:
- Cpl. U.S. Marines.
- Four years in the service of my country.
- Two hitches in Vietnam.
- Five or ten Vietnam War Medals.

> "I used to sleep at the foot of Old Glory,
> And waken to the dawn's early light.

But to my surprise, when I opened my eyes,
I was a victim of the Great Compromise."

Paul B. Payne:
- Lt. Col. USAF (Ret.).
- Thirty years in service.
- WW II Advanced Flight Instructor.
- B-29 Korean War, B-47 from 1953-1959.
- Two years in New Delhi as advisor to Indian Aircraft Industry.
- Participated in two series of atomic tests in Nevada in 1951-1952.
- Vietnam—one year, 1969-1970.

"I have no proof that the government intentionally left Americans behind when we pulled out of Vietnam, but I do believe that the U.S. did leave Southeast Asia knowing that some POWs were still in the hands of the Viet Cong, and our political vacillation was a sure sign of weakness toward winning the conflict.

"It added to Hanoi's determination to demoralize and win an ultimate battle with the U.S. Keeping the POWs was a part of the strategy to eventually cause us to pull out of Vietnam.

"It is difficult to even guess, but many of our WWII, Korean and Vietnam POWs showed extraordinary courage and determination in surviving horrible and barbaric conditions while prisoners. It would not surprise me that some with equal determination are yet alive in Southeast Asia.

"While over there, we should have been allowed to fight to win! Military commanders were the puppets of 'Political Eggheads' and they had no notion that when in a war, you are there to win.

"When our Attorney General and a famous movie actress paraded in the streets of Hanoi in protest to our involvement in the conflict, what conclusions could be drawn but that we were a divided country? I was there when this happened and saw what a devastating effect it had on our troops' morales.

"Little can be done now, but we should continue to press for details for all MIAs.

"My thoughts have changed only to the extent that today we surely see the stupidity that our political experts exhibited in handling the entire conflict."

James P. (Jim) Smith:
- Vietnam Veteran.
- Combat Infantry Badge, National Defense Service Medal, Vietnam Service Medal, Republic of Vietnam Campaign Medal, Republic of Vietnam Meritorious Unit Citation, Armed Forces Expeditionary Medal, Meritorious Unit Commendation Ribbon.
- Fourteen years in the service.

- State Director of the Vietnam Veterans Family Assistance Program.

"I feel strongly that our government did knowingly leave prisoners in Southeast Asia when our forces left. Our government wanted to get out of the war/conflict so badly, a couple thousand men meant nothing to them.

"I feel there are American prisoners still alive. I was in the U.S. Naval Hospital in San Diego, California in 1973 recuperating, when our POWs were released. I was on the third floor and the returning POWs were put on the sixth floor. I had the opportunity to meet most of the ex-POWs and I can tell you some of these men were nothing but shells of men. They were broken both physically and mentally.

"I feel that man's strongest instinct is survival, and if our POWs left over there felt they had been betrayed by their own country, that they may have taken a lifestyle of that country.

"That is why I feel some of our men are still alive. Some of them may have families, and do not want to come back to a country that has turned its back on them, and more than likely would try them for treason.

"The government should have never left there in the first place until we had accounted for all of our men. We should have won the war. The military had the power but the government didn't have the courage and the nation didn't have the will.

"The United States and other countries should keep up the embargo. It seems to have begun to work.

"Twenty to twenty-five years ago, I was full of patriotism, and would have easily laid down my life for this country. After working for years helping veterans from all wars try to get the benefits they have earned, my views of our government have changed greatly. My views about Vietnam have not changed."

Dean Rusk:
- Assistant G-3, General Stilwell's command, New Delhi, India.
- Promoted to full Colonel and received the Legion of Merit with Oak Leaf Cluster.
- Nominated by Gen. Stilwell for Brigadier General but the Pentagon decided the war was drawing to a close and they didn't need any more generals.
- Professor Emeritus of International Law, University of Georgia School of Law.

"I have no information leading to the conclusion that we 'knowingly' left prisoners in Southeast Asia at the time of the Vietnam struggle.

"I think it most unlikely that any Americans who 'might' have been left behind, are still alive today.

"We should have pressed very hard for the return of all Americans, including the remains of such Americans that were dead at the time of the prisoners return. Diplomatic processes cannot be conclusive in such matters, but we should have at least given the matter a good try.

"We should press for a satisfactory accounting on all missing remains of Americans who were taken prisoner during the Vietnam struggle. We should take into account that there have been 'missing in action' in all wars in which the United States has participated, and we cannot guarantee that the process will be satisfactorily concluded.

"With the passage of time, the prospect that there are Americans alive in Vietnam diminishes very rapidly. I would put the emphasis on an accounting for those who have died in Vietnamese hands, but, again, the process cannot be genuinely completed.

"We must face that fact that there will be 'missing in action' who will not be accounted for."

Stanley W. Beesley:
- Vietnam Combat Veteran with the 75th Rangers (First Cavalry and 199th) Light Infantry Brigade.
- Two years in Service.
- LRRP (Long Range Recon. Patrol)—Vietnam and Cambodia.
- Combat Infantry Badge, Bronze Star for Valor.

"Yes, I believe the U.S. government knowingly left prisoners behind in Southeast Asia after 1975. Some were left intentionally for possible covert reasons. Some were left because they had been working on covert operations that had been compromised.

"It seems doubtful that any prisoners are alive. Those few alive will not have been prisoners much beyond 1975. It is my view that these survivors might have willingly assimilated with the captive culture.

"For those legitimate POWs (non-covert operators), I believe much was done to affect their release. MIAs are another issue; I believe little was done on their behalf.

"Our government should now seek to normalize relations with Vietnam. If that poor, ravaged country can forget and forgive us all the pain and misery we visited on their nation, surely a great and powerful land like ours can admit some of our mistakes and go forward.

"This would in no way dishonor the men who fought the American cause, but would establish a dialogue and a political setting which facilitate a Viet-American inquiry and search into the MIA question.

"Think about it: American expertise and technology and Vietnamese tenacity working together in a spirit of cooperation! If there were POWs and MIAs unaccounted for, together we could find them.

"I would go to Vietnam if asked and would be proud to walk the same jungles with men who once tried to kill me and whom I once tried to kill, looking for lost comrades-in-arms. They could show me where they thought Americans fell, and I could show them where Vietnamese fell. That would be a healing process.

"Surprisingly, little of my feelings about the American and my personal experience in Vietnam has changed over the years. A single day does not go by that I do not think of Vietnam and what it meant to my life.

"Silently, at that time, I honor in my small way, every man who fought in that tragic place, both American and Vietnamese. In a perverse sense, the POWs and MIAs have continued serving the American experience in Vietnam.

"The fact that there has been no sensible resolution of their fate has helped to keep the Vietnam War current. This is proper. We should all continue to think of it: for the mistakes that were made and for the honorable efforts expended."

George Plimpton:
- Three and a half years, 752 Tank Bnm. 88th Div.
- Writer/Editor.

"No, I don't think we 'knowingly' left Americans behind when our troops pulled out of Southeast Asia.

"If any are still alive, it would be only those (and mighty few, if any,) who are there on their own volition.

"What should we have done at the time? What time?

"What should we do now? Pretty weird what it has done; a thorough investigation.

"No, my thoughts on Vietnam have not changed over the past 20 years."

Lillis L. (Monte) Waylett:
- Staff Sgt. U.S. Army Artillery (Field Air Assault).
- Batallion Fire Direction and Operations.
- Korea DMZ Skirmishes 1959-1960.
- Nine and a-half years in Service.
- Retired, IBM.

"The issue of POW/MIA has had a very special concern with me. A close schoolmate from National Guard days and a number of troops who worked with me in the Army, went to Vietnam and some never came back. I am still haunted by the last visit of Infantry Captain Bob Carroll who came to see me the day he left for his second tour to Vietnam. He was killed a month later leading an Armored Infantry attack into Cambodia.

"There are so many good, memorable guys, like our gang was. They soldiered with me from 1957 through 1962, and went into combat in Southeast Asia afterward. On three occasions, I have been within 50 yards of the Vietnam Memorial in Washington and have never had guts enough to approach it for fear of finding the names of some very special people on it.

"That is one of the strangest, most forbidding places I have ever found. From an Indian perspective, I can assure anyone that it carries a heap of very potent medicine! I have likewise never attempted to review a list of POW/MIA. I do not think my conscience could take knowing that one of mine might have been left behind. It's bad enough thinking about the people I don't even know.

"Warfare does not bless anyone, blessed are only those who must venture into it. And so it is that you and I love and respect them all. Thank you for what you are doing to show it. In our great society, we reap the rewards of mankind's progress and from this lofty platitude define the word 'civilized'.

"Yet, warfare is the most uncivilized deed any animal could commit upon another. Even though human beings make themselves different from all other beasts by walking upright and covering our feet, I don't think we will be civilized until war is no longer a part of our instincts.

"The POW/MIA issue is a deep, personal dilemma for me. Infantry SFC 'Schultz' Schultzeberger was a D.I. Platoon Sergeant when I met him in 1956 at the USATC, Fort Ord, California. I was then a buck sergeant and assistant D.I., doing my retread stint out of the National Guard, six-months active duty program and back into regular Army.

"Of all the wonderful GIs I have known, I recall my brief association with Schultz as one of the most memorable experiences in life, and to this day wonder where he might be—what might have happened to him.

"I have told his story to many people over the years, people who never realized how much they owed him. Everyone of WWII age owes Schultz a tremendous debt of gratitude because he gave more of his life and energy to his nation's service than anyone I have ever heard of.

"Yet, not a word has ever been written about old Schultz. In the years since that time, the expression 'POW/MIA' has emotionally haunted me with the image of the Schultz I knew back then, the person who taught me more than he knows about the true meaning of freedom, privation and the value of human life and dignity.

"Freedom was taken from Schultz twice in his life, under the most severe circumstances imaginable. For years, every human comfort was denied him, his life continually threatened and his dignity brutalized with each breath he took. Yet with great courage and stamina, he somehow survived to rejoin us in freedom with his undaunted spirit, dignity, immutable character and great sense of humor all in tact. Schultz had achieved a pinnacle of human endurance not unlike the singular ascent of Mount Everest, a feat that most of us would find unimaginable to contemplate—he had survived as a POW (prisoner of war), of two wars.

"When General McArthur was recalled from the Philippines shortly after the outbreak of WWII, Infantry Cpl. Schultzeberger was one of the last hold-outs to be captured by the Japanese at Corregidor Island. Their stiff resistance to the Japanese onslaught had labeled them as dangerous captives even before they were forced to give up and special provisions were made in advance for their imprisonment in Japan.

"After the remnants of his unit were forced into surrender, Schultz and his comrades were loaded into the holds of a cargo ship, destined for an 18-day voyage and internment in Japan. Their prison was a 'compound within a compound' reserved for 'politically incorrigible' prisoners who would be 'specially cared-for' and uniquely isolated from the rest of humanity, especially the prison that surrounded theirs.

"Half the prisoners aboard the ship died in transit, from heat, thirst, starvation and disease. When the voyage started, they were packed in so tightly that there was only room to stand. Rice was thrown down to them once a day through the grated hatches and twice each day water was sprayed on them. When they arrived at port, they were too weak to walk and had to be unloaded with cargo nets, the living in with the dead.

"The stench was so bad that the Japanese had to wear gas masks in order to complete the job. Schultz spent the remainder of the war in that intentionally segregated, most brutal prison camp in Japan. No mail was allowed in or out, no Red Cross, no official accounting of his existence. To the United States, he was MIA.

"Schultz recounted that his repatriation after the war was mostly an alcoholic blur. He had a lot of money saved and spent it all rummaging about the West Coast, thoroughly enjoying his freedom and trying to forget about all his years of pain and deprivation.

"One day he awoke from a drunken stupor in an alley in San Francisco, broke, exhausted and confused, and began wondering how he would ever get up and out of his predicament? All he had ever accomplished of any significance was to become a good soldier at an early age and that was his only occupation.

"So he stumbled around town talking with veterans until he found his way to the recruiting station. He had heard that the services had set up special allowances for the re-enlistment of former POWs and found out that he could join at the rank he held at the time of his capture. He raised his hand again and was happily back in the Army Infantry.

"After several months of medical treatment and rehabilitation, he went back through a refresher training course and was posted to a permanent assignment—back in Japan!

"Schultz wound up as a cadreman at the Camp Zama Army Replacement Center, processing G.I.s in and out of the occupation forces in Japan and Korea. He was there for two years when, in 1950, North Korea crossed the D.M.Z. and invaded South Korea. Business really picked up at the Camp Zama 'repo-depo', but Schultz felt reasonably secure that his permanent job there would remain so.

"Then, just two weeks before a massive U.S. counterattack was to be launched in Korea, Schultz and other permanent party NCO's and officers received orders to draw combat gear and re-qualify with weapons. Afterwards, they were reassigned to combat units and placed on stand-by alert status. Within days, they were loaded onto troop ships and set sail to become part of the invasion at Inchon Bay.

"As Schultz watched flashes of the pre-dawn bombardment of the beachhead from the troop deck of the USS General Mann, he could not believe that he was headed back into a war. He was a squad leader, barely knew the men in his squad and recalled very little about what he should do when he got onto the beach. He said that his whole focus became very simple—'shoot every S.O.B. who looks different and save one for myself if it ever looks like I might get captured!'

"When dawn light was making faint angles through fractures in low rain clouds, Schultz and thousands of others leading the second assault wave were crouched in LST's to avoid pelting rain and salt spray as they churned their way eastward through the heavy mist to land south of Inchon Bay where the Marines were already ashore.

"He found it curious that no one spoke of any counter-fire coming at them and he shuddered to think about the enemy saving it all for a big surprise when they hit the beach. There was visibility of about 100 yards when the ramp crashed down on rock and gravel, and they scrambled up the seawall. Shades of gray outlined cliffs and low ridges that jutted through wisps and pockets of fog and smoke. The naval preparation had advanced inland and its barrage echoed in the distance. No hostile fire could be heard. Maybe this really was 'The Land of the Morning Calm.'

"Orders came to spread out in skirmish formation and advance as far inland as possible. Schultz got his men positioned and moved them out with the standard instruction, 'Follow me.' He recalled that visibility came and went as the morning brightened. The mists formed more densely into scattered pockets and the rain diminished.

"He checked his squad frequently to keep them in sight and in formation. They had not gotten much more than 500 yards inland, when he turned to signal his troops to move up more quickly, and noticed that something looked out of place. As they approached to within a few feet of him, he saw clearly that these troops were wearing soft caps and carring long bayonetted, Japanese-styled rifles! They were on him before he could take another step. He just threw his steel pot onto the ground and shouted, 'Aw S____! Not again!'

"He was bound, gagged, blindfolded and herded into a Korean field compound. From there he was taken north to another Korean POW camp and within a year transferred to a prison camp in China.

"Over the years he was a POW, he escaped twice and was recaptured. Torture and privation were part of everyday survival. But, as Schultz explained it, 'H___, those Koreans and Chinese never even knew the basics of torture when compared to the Japanese. They wrote the book!' Schultz was listed as MIA for two years before the North Koreans named him as a POW. He was one of the last to be repatriated in 1954.

"Now that the story of Sergeant Schultzeberger has been recounted, one might understand the impact his tales of prisoner life had upon another attentive and respectful young soldier. This is small tribute for all he endured and the least I could do to settle part of the debt he has earned.

"Moreover, one cannot think of the ordeals of this man without having a very special concern for anyone who has ever become a prisoner of war. So it has been with me—a deep and earnest concern for those lost to the enemy.

"I, for one, have never forgotten what they sacrificed to fight our nation's battles. It has also been almost unbearable to think that our nation might have knowingly forsaken anyone who might have become a prisoner of our enemies in Vietnam. Schultz told me without blinking an eye, that in every day he was a POW he derived strength from absolute confidence that his country would do anything to bring him home once it was all over. And so he committed to his survival.

"When I had the enemy on my firing charts along the Korean DMZ, they also had me plotted. Duels broke out and stealthy patrols penetrated our defenses. People were killed and wounded. We took prisoners and gave up none that I knew of. But the possibility of becoming a prisoner was there for all of us and we all trusted that we could survive, believing for certain that our country would never leave us behind when the battles were over.

"The epilogue of the Vietnam war has left me with bitter feelings about such beliefs and an anxiety that never subsides about our nation's conscience and principles. Were our warriors forsaken in that war? Did our government know and not diligently pursue every effort to get them out? Did the government try to cover-up its failures by deceit and denial?

"I am shamed to admit that, in my personal opinion, the answer to all of these questions is 'yes'. I do not admit this lightly. I became concerned about POW/MIAs when we first became engaged in Vietnam. I participated in the first Army adaptations of helicopter air assault and fire support base concepts when I was with the 4th Infantry Division (STRAC) at Fort Lewis, Washington.

"I remember how unreal it seemed to me at the time that a light artillery battery could even think of occupying a position that was not defended by at least a regiment of infantry. Hell, when you have cannons or heavy mortars to shoot, it just doesn't seem natural to have to drop everything, jump up and chase the enemy around camp with pistols and carbines.

"But, that's about what it seems was intended and the way it worked out. Disadvantage—losses, and many of them POW/MIA! The whole idea had a lot of 'pucker' in it for me and that's what has made me sensitive about seeing the names on the long stone wall of the memorial. But they died as soldiers and sailors must in war. They were honored and are remembered and their spirits walk nobly among us. What about those who still have not come home, their honored places empty and their tributes unpaid?

"When the organization, Operation Skyhook, was first formed, I became a charter member. At the time, there was every reason to believe that we had left military people behind in Vietnam, Laos and Cambodia. I had revulsion over thoughts that our government might have intentionally covered-up the real circumstances of POW/MIAs and I did not believe enough had been done to recover them.

"At the time, the defense department had listed some 2,300 service people as MIA after the president's assurances that all of our POWs had been returned. Therefore, my first question in a letter to Skyhook was about the estimated 2,000 military deserters living in the bowels of Saigon at the time that U.S. forces pulled out.

"'Did the organization's objective of determining the circumstances of 2,300 MIAs include the same 2,000 who were listed as deserters? If so, don't include me if they were going to attempt to get them back. They don't deserve any more than they chose. On the other hand, if deserters are not part of the objective, count me in.' I never heard from Skyhook again, and understand that it was probably some kind of scam anyhow.

"In recent months, I have had the opportunity to watch most of the U.S. Senate's Select Committee on POW/MIA hearings on C-SPAN. At their conclusion, I assessed the effort as one deserving the highest respect and praise, and said so in a letter to Senator Kerry. I do not think I have ever seen an element of our elected government act so intently, thoroughly and earnestly on any subject within the limited time they had to deal with such a complex and well-defended issue.

"I expected that if their efforts found the truth, it would not sit well with America. They found the truth and didn't avoid anything in explaining what they found. If the 'truth shall set us free,' then perhaps their report will substantiate for our future, all the wrongs that were done that allowed our country to forsake our POW/MIAs, so that this country will never repeat them.

"Our government did know that there were POW/MIAs in Laos long after president Nixon assured the nation that all Vietnam War POWs were returned or accounted for. We were subjected to a terrible lie in favor of political expediency.

"Ross Perot reported that there were '10s of 10s' of American prisoners in the hands of the Laotian military after the war and that no one had officially asked about negotiating for their return. The simplest course was to label them 'MIAs,' forget about them and prevent anyone else from discovering them.

"How many were there? No one knows. No centralized records are kept by the Laotians and we have no political or economic basis to exert any influence with their government to determine what prisoners they may have had.

"Laos is a stone wall to our investigators and there is no present avenue around it. Is there any possibility that any prisoners could have survived until now? Doubtful. Their discovery would be a tremendous liability to their captors and they could never have represented much more than slave labor assets.

"In all probability, they died of privation or were intentionally killed to prevent discovery. Yet, recalling the singular element that kept Schultz' spirit alive, our comrades may have at some time concluded that their country had given up on them. Their spirits suffered this final degradation and they died of broken hearts.

"By now, their eradication would be as complete as is humanly possible. Today, the attitude of the Laotian government is in full accord with the position of the Nixon administration—'After the war, those people never existed.'"

Raymond Q. Swanson:
- POW WWII Veteran with the 44th Combat Engineers.
- U.S. Army for two years, 10 months and 13 days.
- POW Medal, Purple Heart with two Oak Leaf Clusters, EAME Campaign Medal with five Bronze Stars, Croix de Guerre-France.

"I was captured in Germany on December 19, 1944, and was liberated on May 28, 1945. I wish I could help on the MIA situation in Southeast Asia.

"Our government should have done so many things about finding and bringing back POWs in Southeast Asia at the time when the war was over. Our government has been trying to forget about the POWs there for the last 18 years."

Jimmie R. Duffield:
- Vietnam Veteran, 101st Airborne. 25th Infantry Division.
- Two Bronze Stars with Oak Leaf Clusters.

"I don't think we knowingly left any POW/MIAs and I don't know if any are still alive if they were left, but, we should have stayed over there until we were sure.

"Right now, we should go back over there and get a full accounting of Americans. My thoughts haven't changed about Vietnam in the past 20 years but I hear you can now go back over there as a tourist and travel all those places we used to fight for. I don't know about that."

Warren B. Henry:
- U.S. Navy. Four years in Vietnam.

"Yes, we did leave Americans behind when the U.S. Forces pulled out of Southeast Asia in 1975.

"Probably, there are some still alive over there.

"The U.S. government should have stayed and fought with both hands.

"Now, the government should tell the truth and force the enemy, through economic and political means, to release our prisoners and records.

"My thoughts haven't changed, we could have won the war!"

James (Jim) Ogletree:
- Col. U.S. Army (Ret.).
- Thirty-three years and nine months service.
- WWII Battery Commander, 564th Field Artillery, 71st Infantry Division, Patton's 3rd Army.

"Did we knowingly leave people over there when our forces pulled out is a very difficult question. I'm sure we knowingly did, but did we deliberately leave them? You have to understand that in a combat area like that, in that kind of country, you will have dead people in the jungle that you'll never find or even know what happened to them.

"A platoon Sergeant comes back in from a patrol, a fierce firefight, especially a night fight, and there are some guys missing. The last time they were seen was trying to get over to the flank or to assist a wounded comrade and the fighting forced a 'pull back' and they are never seen again. You can't get around that sort of thing.

"The U.S. was in a rout to get out of there. It was the most disgusting thing ever, in any way, shape or form. Who would know what happened to our troops in a retreat like that. I don't think the enemy was in hot pursuit, we were running from the pressure put on the military by it's own government and especially college students. It took a long time to check your people in a retreating situation. It never made any sense at all.

"I doubt if anyone is still alive if they were left. Given the extreme cruelty the Vietnamese were known for. It's just been too long for anyone to survive in a POW situation. In some easier situations, sure, some might have survived and even still be alive today, but no way could they have survived in POW conditions.

"What should we have done at the time? The President couldn't even figure out what to do! We left there in chaos with no surrender agreement of any kind. We ran, they didn't pursue us. So, how could we have 'gone back?' We were on the run. We couldn't have started the fighting and the combat and the bombing back up again. We were 'pulling out!' It's just that simple.

"We've exhausted every available clue. I know it's painful to the families but what these people need to know is that the U.S. government had no will to win this war. The American citizens had no will to keep fighting. The soldier was very confused by the orders to fight and all the time hearing how the Americans back home were against what they were doing.

"The soldiers did what they were told to do. There was just no emphasis from Washington that they wanted to win this war. The soldiers always did what they were told to do. They just didn't have the support of America.

"An Army Sergeant in a helicopter unit told me they had an LZ (landing zone) close to a Vietnamese village. They received orders that they were not permitted to fire into the villages.

"Well, what kind of war have you got here? The enemy had no uniforms, they wore the same things the civilians wore and what did they do? Sure, they went right into the villages and opened up on the U.S. Army LZ with automatic rifles and mortar shells but the Americans could not fire back. The enemy knew this too.

"The commander called in for permission to return fire at noon but by 4:00 p.m. had not received the go-ahead and lost every single U.S. Army helicopter, the gasoline storage and all their equipment and most of the men.

"When you're trying to fight a war like that, you've got it lost before you start. Morale goes and the soldiers soon say, 'What the heck, we're not allowed to shoot back and we're getting shot up.' It was a terrible situation.

"Advisers asked Washington, 'How bad do you want to win this war?' Possibly if President Kennedy had lived he would have gotten us out.

Everyone laughed at McGovern but all he was saying was, 'We'll never win that thing over there with this much American dissension so we might as well get out of it before we lose any more lives.'

"We might as well forget it and write off the POW/MIAs. You know the American public were the very ones who were yelling to get the troops out. Now, they say get the troops back in there and account for our POW/MIAs. There's no way.

"The only way to get an accounting of at least the ones we knew for sure were POWs, is to go back to war and start bombing Hanoi into oblivion. Well, do you really think the American public is ready to go back to Vietnam and start the war up again? No! The American public has to share the blame for the POW/MIA situation. It is the fault of our government who did not have the will or courage to fight an all-out war against a viscious enemy as American soldiers ever faced.

"But, still they asked the soldiers to fight and die while they pondered how to get out. But, it is just as much the fault of the American citizen and the college students who criticized everything the military did. They have to take the blame for some of this.

"Boy, we needed a man like Gen. Patton over there. He didn't beat around the bush, he came to the punch each time. However, had he had the dissension from the college students and the public like the military leaders during Vietnam did, he might not have been so great.

"But, he had a loving American public behind him and no college student dissension. They stood up for their military leaders back then and kept their mouths shut. If they weren't fighting the war, they sure didn't beat down those who were with a lot of crying and talking.

"So, students and the general public have to shoulder some of the blame for leaving POW/MIAs behind. They forced their own government to hurry and get out without a clear-cut victory. Let them face their concience. It's partly their fault and I hope they are proud of their actions. It cost an awful lot of American lives.

"My Artillery Battery was on the move one night and I lead them through the narrow streets of a small German village. My jeep driver turned a corner and almost had a head-on collision with General Patton and his jeep driver.

"We came to attention and saluted and Gen. Patton yelled, 'Get that G–D– jeep out of the way and let a fighting S.O.B. through here.' Our battery pulled over and let his outfit pass. Yeah, we needed more like Patton over there. With American support, of course."

John F. Sommer, Jr.:
- Executive Director of the American Legion–1.3 million members.

"Various forms of evidence have been shared with the American Legion by families and interested individuals which lead us to believe that live prisoners are being held in Southeast Asia.

"No government official or entity can, or will, say for certain whether any American POWs are still alive in captivity; however, based on the evidence we have reviewed we believe there are live prisoners in Southeast Asia. In any case, the U.S. government should do everything reasonably possible to make an absolute determination, and to address the situation accordingly.

"We have specified some of the actions that the U.S. government should have taken in the past and should take in the future to keep faith with personnel in the armed forces and their families.

"It has become apparent that individuals within the government who are charged with the responsibility of accounting for our POW/MIAs have not done their jobs, and in some cases have expended more effort at damage control than analysis and investigation of live prisoners of war.

"Real progress on the POW/MIA issue depends upon active work like that which you are doing, so we are pleased to learn of your personal commitment on the vitally important POW/MIA issue."

Charles H. "Chief" Horner:
- 877th Airborne. Glider Pilot.
- Combat Engineers, Co A.
- Three years in the Service.

"We traveled in gliders. We did numbers of things during WWII, but were promised a lot of things but never received anything.

"I am just thankful to be at home and writing to you. The POW/MIA issue is very dear to my heart. I have friends who were POWs.

"After what the American soldier has gone through for our government, I just hope our government will not give in to Vietnam until our POW/MIAs are accounted for."

Dan Lewis:
- Vietnam Veteran. E-5, five years, three months, 26 days service.
- HHC 3rd Bn. 22nd Infantry, 4th Division.
- HHC 3rd Bde. 25th Infantry Division.
- Radio Retrans. (Infantry) Remote Outposts, Long Range.
- Vietnam Service Medals, Unit Presidential Citations, Bronze Star, Combat Infantry Badge.
- "Operations in Country" and battles include, Iron Triangle, Attleboro, Junction City, Gadsden, Firebase Gold, Soi Rte., French Fort, Nui Ba Dcn (Black Virgin Mountain), Soi Da, Cu Chi.

- Past Commander of American Legion Post #50.

"Soldiers don't leave soldiers . . . Politicians leave soldiers.

"I believe the government did leave POW/MIAs intentionally, partly due to the expansion of the combat role into Cambodia and Laos. And, the possibility that many covert operations were taking place then and the years following the war.

"It is very likely some could possibly still be alive considering how long our returning POWs survived in Vietnamese captivity.

"We should not have left Vietnam until all POW/MIAs were accounted for, or a reasonable doubt as to their existence or last known wherebouts.

"Today, we should negotiate more with the Vietnamese—now that Vietnam is open to U.S. travel. But, are these (POWs U.S. Military) that fought in the war?

"Perhaps they are 'captives' of other motives, soldiers of fortune, CIA, or opportunists. However, we must never leave our Military POW/MIAs or stop trying to free them.

"The first 20 years after Vietnam I would not have thought the U.S. would leave any POWs or stop trying to locate MIAs. But, after Agent Orange and other cover-ups and deceptions the fighting soldiers have experienced, I firmly believe the whereabouts of soldiers, whether in Vietnam, Cambodia, Laos, China or Russia, is known by the Vietnamese officials. So, should we lift the embargo?

"The United States must never abandon its combat veterans. Whether it be on home soil or on the battlefield. These are a special breed of men that love their country and are willing to die for it.

"Every veteran should live in dignity, knowing their country will care for them as they cared for their country. God bless us all."

George Koch:
- Korean War Veteran. U.S. Army Airborne/Ranger. (Ret.)
- Served in Korea with 75 Rangers, 3rd Bn. Co. B. Made three combat jumps with the 187th R.C.T. (Regimental Combat Team). Served with 7th Infantry Division, Special Operations.
- Combat Infantry Badge, Purple Heart, Silver Star, Bronze Star, two Presidential Unit Citations, Korean Presidential Unit Citation, two Campaign Ribbons with Star, 17 Ribbons.

"Yes, we knowingly left POW/MIAs in Southeast Asia when our troops pulled out.

"Yes, some of those prisoners are still alive.

"At the time of withdrawal, the U.S. government should have achieved greater military superiority to afford the enemy an absolute 'No Victory' status.

"We should have bombed North Vietnam more aggressively in order to de-moralize the enemy population and force their government to negotiate prisoner exchange and accountability.

"Today, our government should refuse to recognize North Vietnam and intensify our embargo on all goods, humanitarian or otherwise, until they make an honest effort to account for **all** POW/MIAs.

"My thoughts concerning Vietnam have not changed at all during the past 20 years."

David Boren:
• United States Senator, Washington, D.C.

"The POW/MIA issue is one of great importance to me. Accounting for the missing from the Vietnam conflict has been a priority during my chairmanship of the Senate Intelligence Committee.

"I co-sponsored the initiative to establish the select POW/MIA Committee in the Senate which recently ended its investigation and will soon issue its final report for distribution.

"The report will undoubtedly hold answers to many questions. Another success is the passage of Senator McCain's bill, which I also co-sponsored, to declassify as much information as possible concerning the POW/MIAs.

"The new cooperation between Washington and Hanoi has made it possible for a new 50-member U.S. Defense Department Joint Task Force to conduct investigations of sighting reports in Vietnam.

"We are pressing the Vietnamese who have begun to keep their promise to let us research their military archives. These files contain information not only about losses in Vietnam, but also in Laos and Cambodia where the Vietnamese military controlled the battlefields.

"I hope and pray that with all of these new opportunities we can finally achieve the fullest possible accounting of all those who are missing in Southeast Asia."

Robert L. Marks:
• WWII. Co. I 290th Infantry, 75th Division.
• Korea. Co F. 19th Infantry, 24th Division.
• Bronze Star, Purple Heart with Cluster, 2nd Award of Combat.
• Infantryman's Badge, six Bronze Battle Stars, (Korea 4, E.T.O. 2), Good Conduct Medal, Meritorious Unit Citation (24th Div.), several Campaign Ribbons and Marksmanship Awards.

"I should preface my comments by stating that I was never a Prisoner of War but I am acquainted with men who were. One of them, our Company Commander's radio man, was captured by the Germans near St. Vith, Belgium in early 1945 during the Battle of the Bulge.

"Two of them were Air Force personnel shot down over Germany. One of my acquaintances was captured on Corregidor with General Wainwright and was held captive on the mainland of Japan for the remainder of WWII.

"The thoughts I have to offer are primarily opinions and impressions based on conversations with these men, my own personal experiences in Belgium and Korea, some of the reading I have done, and radio and television coverage.

"I am sure it is quite possible that some Americans were taken to Russia, as alleged in articles in *Soldier of Fortune* magazine, family members, congressional and veterans groups, but how authentic they are, I really do not know.

"Knowing the ruthlessness with which Stalin often operated, it would not surprise me at all if it was proven that some of the assertions by Sanders, Kirkwood and Sauter were really true as mentioned in their story, 'Forsaken in the Gulag,' in an issue of the *New American*.

"If men were taken to Russia under these circumstances it probably was an effort on their part to obtain classified military information. After all, Russia, for a long time, has not been a close friend of the United States. Frankly, I think it behooves us to keep our 'powder dry' because there are still lots of hard-core Communists in Russia.

"From my experiences in the early Army of Occupation of Germany at the close of WWII, conversation between GIs at that time, and reading books by General Bradley and Eisenhower, I doubt seriously that any Americans were kept in Germany against their will.

"It seems reasonable to assume that we did lose many men in concentration camps primarily due to very poor living conditions and cruel, psychological treatment. Some of the latter inflicted by German civilians, adults and children alike, during lengthy, forced marches, usually at night.

"A great many Americans were taken prisoner in Korea, especially in the summer and fall months of 1950. My own Infantry Division, the 24th, was hit very hard with these losses. It is alleged that many of these prisoners were taken to Russia. I suspect that was true since the Russians were so involved politically and militarily in the Korean conflict.

"Our outfit saw and felt quite a bit of Russian armament before, during and after my tenure in Korea. After I returned home in September of 1951, I kept up with the negotiations in Panmunjom regarding the settlement of hostilities.

"The exchange of prisoners was a gut-wrenching, lengthy affair with the Koreans. No doubt, the Chinese and Russian governments played a big role in the repatriation of prisoners on both sides. However, bear in mind that there were a few prisoners involving governments of a few other countries as well.

"It does not take a great deal of imagination to think that a few GI's may have been lost due to combat death and the inability of our forces to recapture their bodies.

"It is my visceral feeling that some of those American prisoners taken prisoner in Korea were simply buried or left in the mountains and no record kept of their burial places. Though these events are sometimes facts of Infantry combat, they do not diminish the grief and loss suffered by the families of missing men.

"I have no factual knowledge of American Prisoners of War having been kept by either China or Russia but if it suited their needs at the time, I would not doubt it at all. It is my belief that our government, under the circumstances, did about all they could to close the Korean War and retrieve as many of our missing men as was possible.

"We did not prosecute that conflict as forcefully as we should have because too many politicians in Washington, Seoul, Pyongyang, Peking, and Moscow got in the way. Thus, some bitterness lingers yet today in the minds of many ex-GIs and civilians as well.

"Of course, our biggest dilemma concerning the returning of Prisoners of War came about during the Vietnam conflict. The war we failed to allow our troops to win! Presidents Kennedy and Johnson, I believe, were too inept in their decisions.

"They allowed too many disheveled, morally corrupt, hell-raisers with a sad lacking of commitment to freedom from communism—too big a role in formulating public opinion. Many civilians and people in government at that time also suffered from a lack of backbone.

"We should have untied the hands of our armed forces and taken charge of the land mass of Vietnam rather than leave in an emergency situation with so many loose ends left untied. We could have accounted for many more of our POW/MIAs and burial sites which could have been exhumed.

"It seems inconceivable to me that any member of our armed forces would elect to stay in Vietnam which causes me to suspect that most of those we lost were simply buried by the enemy in some unmarked spot which probably will never be found.

"Some may have been left because of the nature of intense combat situations. I doubt that it was always possible to retrieve bodies of fallen comrades.

"We should continue as long as it takes to get every piece of information concerning our POW/MIAs. That will have to be done by the proper people in governments and not by politicians seeking political gain as they so often want to do.

"I hardly believe that our government knowingly and deliberately deserted POW/MIAs, but I suppose it is possible knowing the shenanigans that some governmental officials have undertaken in other endeavors. Not meaning to be overly critical or cynical of politicians in general, but we have always been plagued by too many who lack that patriotic 'fire in the belly' required when the best interests of our union are at stake. Ultimately, these responsibilities rest, as they should, on the shoulders of our electorate which is why voters should always keep the sanctity of our country in mind, for as Daniel Webster wrote: 'God grants liberty only to those who love it and are always ready to guard and defend it.'

"As I have grown older, I suppose my opinions have mellowed somewhat with respect to some military decisions that were made in our assaults that, at the time, should have been done differently.

"After all, our leaders at the time were also younger and not infallible. Though I did not serve in Vietnam, I still have misgivings about the lack of support of our nation offered our forces. Authorities of the national and local level should not have tolerated so much riotous disorder in the streets and on college campuses. Students were abetted and allowed too much leeway in there and (there was) destruction of class and buildings.

"Courts and governmental officials permitted them entirely too much concern for their freedoms and too little for their responsibilities with thousands of their young generation leaking out their blood in Vietnam fighting Communism. Too much of our nations's life blood and energies was wasted on too many acts of rebelliousness. This, from a generation of young people, many of whom were raised in homes of affluency."

William C. Anderson:
- WWII Bomber Pilot, Flew Berlin Airlift, Flew Hurricanes for the AWS, Flew Air Evac. in Korea, Served in Pentagon—the bloodiest battle of all—for four years. Visited Vietnam upon Air Force Retirement as War Correspondent.
- Usual collection of medals and citations.
- Wrote several military books and screenplays such as "Bat-21."

"To my knowledge, no prisoners were left in Asia knowingly and none are still alive, unless they have chosen to remain in Vietnam of their own volition.

"Our government was not remiss in its duties at the time, and it has done everything within its power since.

"All the POW/MIAs will never be accounted for, just as we still have missing soldiers from previous wars.

"It's time to close the book on the POWs and get on with our lives."

Hubert E. Wilson:
- U.S. Navy: 20 years in the Service with two Battle Stars.
- Vietnam Veteran.

"Yes, I think we left several there.

"I personally think they were alive for years, but I do believe that most are gone now except a few that elected to stay there on their own.

"At the end of the war, we should have gone in and got them regardless of the cost or public opinion.

"I used to think that all resources should be used to get them out, but now I believe it would be a waste of time and resources to even try to get the remains. We would undoubtedly have to pay for the help and we really wouldn't know if what we get is the real thing. Vietnam is not known for their honesty.

Alex Borowski:
- M/Sgt. (Ret.) 173rd 82nd Airborne.
- Fifteen years in Service.
- Bronze Star with Cluster, Vietnam Gallantry Cross with Palm Cluster, Nominated for Silver Star in 1968.

"Yes, POWs were left in Southeast Asia when our troops pulled out in 1973. They were sold out by Washington. (Expendable.)

"It is doubtful any are still alive. Most were executed or died of dreadful conditions.

"What our government should have done back then was had a full accounting by on-site inspectors prior to our withdrawal.

"What we should do now is increase sanctions until we are positive that the NVA is truthful.

"The only way my thoughts have changed over the past 20 years is the possibility of live Americans being found."

Bennett M. Guthrie II:
- Vietnam Veteran. 1st Cavalry Division. 1 Bde. (Airborne).
- 2nd Bn. 8th Cavalry 1965-1966.
- Vietnam Cross of Gallantry with Palm, CIB, Parachute Wings.
- Presidential Unit Citation four times, Army Commendation Medal, Air Medal, Army Achievement Medal, Humanitarian Service, Vietnam Campaign Medal, Service, etc.

"I have the gut feeling that the government left POW/MIAs behind when our forces pulled out of Vietnam.

"The government has its own way of dealing with situations. They usually tell the public one thing while doing something else."

Jerold M. Starr:
  • Director, Center for Social Studies Education, Pittsburgh.

"I do not believe that the U.S. government knowingly left prisoners in Vietnam when our forces left. Whether covert operatives were abandoned in Laos is still open to question. A lot of Americans were lost in Laos.

"Certainly, our government should always seek the fullest accounting possible for U.S. servicemen MIA, acknowledging, of course, the serious limitations of such investigation.

"I believe that goal would best be achieved today by normalizing diplomatic relations with Vietnam, Laos and Cambodia and encouraging trade and travel.

"The more Americans permitted to travel and live in Southeast Asia, the greater the chance of being able to resolve more cases."

George Edward Boggs:
  • WWII. Capt. USMCR. Marine Aircraft Group 12, VMF-211 Korea. VMF-235. F4U Corsairs, both wars.
  • Flew in John Wayne movie, "Flying Leathernecks."
  • Distinguished Flying Cross, five Air Medals, Presidential Unit Citation, Asiatic Pacific, Navy Unit Citation, China Service Medal, American Theater Ribbon, Philippine Liberation Medal, WWII Victory Medal, National Defense Service Medal, 1055-E (Experience Fighter Pilot,) Flew off USS Sicily in Korea, Close Air Support & Combat Air Patrol.

"We did not leave any POW/MIAs from my unit. I think there may be some POW/MIAs still alive from the Vietnam War left in Southeast Asia, especially Laos and Cambodia.

"I wish to suggest to you a fine story about Lorin Grised of Santa Ana, California. Lorin became MIA during WWII and it affected my own life a lot because I was acquainted with his father who expressed extreme faith in the Lord at that very time. Popo said to me at church, 'Lorin is missing in action,' and with a tear in his eye said, 'The Lord is with Lorin.'

"My own faith was strengthened. Lorin's story is a good one and a condensed version of his story is written in *It Takes Two To Untangle Tongues* by Ethel Emily Wallis 1985, available from Wycliffe Bible Translators, Hunington Beach, CA. Lorin has been successful in the insurance field and has been the Mayor of Santa Ana a couple of times. A fine Christian and friend and gives God the Glory!

"We did lose some men from our unit VMF 211 in the Philippines in WWII. I don't remember any of the men being taken prisoner. Lt. Brown had to ditch and I circled him for some time until a rescue craft (Dumbo) appeared on the scene.

"In Korea, we searched for a missing plane for several hours, but we could not locate him at all. I can't recall the pilot's name now. One of our planes shot down a MIG-15 with a piston engine plane, an F4U Corsair. A lot of excitement that day. Jess Fuller was shot down a few days later but was rescued with some serious injuries after he bailed out.

"I don't think there is much our government can do about POW/MIAs that have been missing for so many years. Console families perhaps. Perhaps a few have chosen Asian culture to live and have families there now and simply did not want to come home."

James R. Wagner:
- POW Korean Veteran. Hospital Corpsman serving with U.S. Marine Corps. 1951-1955.
- POW exchange- "Freedom Village" both "Operation Little Switch" and "Operation Big Switch."
- American Legion National Chaplain.

"If we knowingly left POW/MIAs, definition is important—did we 'purposely' leave some behind? No! Did we know there were some unaccounted for? Probably! Even, Yes! Was it intended to leave them? NO! They probably thought exchange and release would be secured by diplomatic means.

"When that didn't work—the issue went to 'back burner' status—then, when we 'woke up'—confusion, misinformation, etc. took over to keep the situation clouded—as it is now.

"If any are still alive? There may be a few, however, I have an idea that most are probably dead as results of wounds, execution, starvation, etc.

"We should never enter a conflict without the intention of victory. Therefore, we should have made sure of the release potential before our withdrawal.

"Now, the government should make a last ditch, all-out, thorough investigation, on site, settle once and for all, with complete, one-for-one accounting, based on actual POW/MIA list.

"No! My thoughts have not changed concerning Vietnam the past 20 years.

"This is a high-priority matter affecting the morale of the nation and servicemen. Especially, the government should give their best effort so our military personnel will never again be confronted with the appearance of not caring."

Thomas H. Taylor:
- Author: *Where The Orange Blooms*.
- Vietnam Veteran with 2-502, 1st Bde. 101st Airborne (1965-1966).
- Eight years in the military.
- Silver Star, Bronze Star with Valor and Oak Leaf Cluster, Purple Heart.

"First, enclosed is the only information concerning POW/MIAs which I've firsthand knowledge. It comes from my book, *Where The Orange Blooms.*

"'. . . he said, yeah, they even have some air photos of that.' I asked him if Americans thought that was counterrevolution, but he did not want to discuss this with me.

"Mostly Hai Bach was interested in U.S. MIAs. 'Only thing I know is in Long Trang, 1975 or 1976, cadre said they kept some U.S. troops for trade for U.S. aid. They said this with other bull s— about how strong and important SVR is in the world. I don't know if this is true about MIAs—a lot of people ask me. Everything cadre told us was lies. If they (still) have MIAs it would be the only true thing they ever said.

"'Nobody I ever met saw any Americans in Vietnam since 1975. The war was over in 1973. If any are still there, they are kept in the north. Personally, I don't think there are any more POWs alive. Maybe some AWOL GIs married Vietnamese and accept life there, but I never heard about anyone like that either.'

"Hai Bach wanted to know everything like this. If there are Caucasians around. How do we know they are French? They said the Viet Minh kept some French Officers.

"Hai Bach said there were war rumors that NVA kept some POWs to do maintenance on modern American equipment. He asked if that makes sense to me. 'This is a possibility. Maybe in the Air Force this happens. When I hid around the waterfront, I saw ships loading U.S. airplane parts . . . .'

"As of this date, the Kerry Committee is generating more information than has been available for decades. Their tentative conclusion (as yet unpublished) seems to answer the first question: Yes, we did knowingly leave POWs behind in Laos. Which is to say we did not lean hard enough on Hanoi to force their Pathet Lao puppets to release the POWs they held. I doubt very much if any are now living. Unless . . . their captors (wanted) to preserve them. Prison conditions would have killed them within 10 years. I believe the last one died in 1980. (That is seven years after the government said none were alive.) For a hair-raising description of captivity under the Pathet Lao, read *Escape From Laos.*

"I've spoken with MIA wives who believe their men would have been preserved for their technical knowledge. And it would have been Hanoi who would have wanted them; the Pathet Lao were too primitive. I imagine that Hanoi sent Tech Reps. to interview every Airman captured by the Pathet Lao. We should lean heavily on Hanoi to determine if they did, and who they saw, and the POW's condition. Even now, Hanoi has considerable leverage on Laos. We should insist on the return of remains from Laos. Hanoi can get them.

"Precedence from WWII and Korea indicate that our government is prepared to write off POW/MIAs. A recent *20/20* (ABC) piece on this subject corroborates. Tom Jarrel was the reporter.

"On a personal level, the fate of our MIAs appalls me. Administrations back to LBJ refused to tell the American people the facts. To send a guy into combat was like writing him a one-way ticket if he was captured.

"Perhaps this is cynical, but if Hanoi had never revealed they held POWs, we never would have insisted that they be returned. And, incidentally, the Son Tay Raid might never have been attempted–Gen. Risner can tell you how important the raid was for the POWs–because then, no matter if the raid was successful or not, the government would have had to admit that there were POWs.

"The only upside from our Vietnam experience in this matter was our policy regarding POWs in Iraq during the Gulf War. Gen. Powell made it crystal clear that there would be a full accounting from Baghdad or the war would continue. We got everybody back (and that included every body, too.) This is the only way we should ever end a war.

"I'm confident that because of our Vietnam experience, the POW/MIA Issue continues as an important consideration in foreign policy. No doubt, when reviewing the consequences of intervention in Yugoslavia, the Pentagon asked the State Department what we'd do if one of the factions captured some of our servicemen? Who would we deal with for their release? How could we track down MIAs? These questions are like velcro when the government tries to move toward decisions. That's good. The American public is sensitized to POW/MIAs as never before in our history. Our Military martyrs from the Vietnam War have made this so.

"The MIA families are equally Martyrs—even more, I think. The MIAs died but once, but their survivors lived on, tortured by uncertainty, denied even the grim outcome of finality. They received lip service from the government in return for the ultimate service their loved ones performed for their Country. God owes them a special mercy for a debt from America that can never be paid on earth. May there be a joyous reunion in the life to come.

"A photo taken of Ben Cai Lam and MG (now LTG) Binnie Peay, CG of the 101st Airborne in the Gulf War, when standing together at The Wall, seems a bridge between two wars, one as depressing as the other was triumphant."

Carl T. Reichert:
- 1st Air Cav. Division. (January 1968-June 1968).
- 577th Engineer Bn. (July 1968-December 1968).

"I thought then and continue to believe that our Country was wrong to turn its back on the fate of our missing servicemen.

"We should never have left Vietnam while questions concerning the whereabouts of our comrades remained unanswered or answers to these questions remained unverified."

John A. Ketcher:
- Deputy Principal Chief-Cherokee Nation of Oklahoma.
- U.S. Navy—U.S.S. New Orleans, 1943-1946.
- Fourteen Battle and Engagement Stars.

"I have no concrete facts to substantiate stories that the United States deliberately or knowingly left forces captured or to be captured by the North Vietnamese. But . . . if the enemy 'was' holding our servicemen when we pulled out, then . . . there is a strong possibility we did leave some men behind.

"The details of the disengagement allude me after 20 years and I do not remember the facts of the withdrawal. Whether our leaving was tied to their releasing American servicemen, I do not recall.

"There is enough difference in physical appearance of Americans that it would be difficult to hide anyone in Vietnam for any length of time. However, Laos would be a different story."

John Reid III:
- First Bn. 3rd Marines, Vietnam 1967-1968.
- Fifth Communications Bn. Vietnam 1969-1970.
- Two Vietnam Tours totaling 25 months.
- Radio-Telegraph Operator-Artillery & Naval Gunfire FO.
- Participated in 29 Combat Operations as part of Special Landing Force between April 1967 and December 1967.
- Received Combat Action Ribbon, Naval Unit Citation, Presidential Unit Citation & Republic of Vietnam Unit Awards.

"A full accounting of the deaths of those listed as MIAs should be obtained from whatever sources possible."

Lee Rutledge:
- WWII U.S. Navy Diver.
- Bronze Star, Pearl Harbor. Rescued 32 from sunken U.S.S. Oklahoma.

"I retired from the U.S. Navy in 1954, so I have no knowledge of anything about the Vietnam War. I would not, could not, understand any government that would leave members of the Armed Forces deserted. If it is ever proven though, we should dig up their graves, etc."

William D. Armer:
- Two years in Vietnam with 442 Transportation Co.

"Yes, I think we did in fact leave behind Americans in Southeast Asia when our troops pulled out.

"I still believe there are some of them alive today.

"We had the Forces to get them out at the time but thanks to our government, we did not.

"In my opinion, this is a disgrace to the Vietnam Veterans."

Dennis Hannah:
- WWII 82nd Airborne Division. 1942-1945.
- Silver Star, Bronze Star, Purple Heart, etc. Battle of Normandy. Served in European Theater of Operation.

"I feel that I cannot answer questions as I did not serve in Southeast Asia . . . however . . . if prisoners were left behind when our troops withdrew in 1973, I feel that every effort should be made to bring them home."

John G. Pribram:
- WWII Medic with 254th Inf. 63rd Div.
- Silver Star, Purple Heart, Combat Medical Badge.
- Military experiences are recalled in my book, *Horizons of Hope,* page 28-33.
- Educator (Ret.) and Author.

"As you probably notice, I did not fight in the Vietnam War, I never visited Asia and my knowledge of this area of operation is extremely limited. I was a prisoner myself at one time. I escaped Nazi occupation as a young boy on a bicycle and on a freighter bound for the United States.

"I was educated in the U.S. then on to Harvard, then into the U.S. Army where I was sent back to Europe to fight the Nazis in my very own country.

"Concerning the possibility of knowingly leaving POWs in Southeast Asia, I hope we did not.

"I do not think that some of the prisoners are still alive.

"The government should have been more alert and put pressure on Vietnam to release prisoners, once we were aware of a POW/MIA.

"The government is doing the right thing now, by sending various officials to Vietnam and discovering more documents and even remains of POW/MIAs.

"The more one discovers, the more one gets concerned about what's going on with the POW/MIA Issue."

Donovan Hamilton:
- WWII Veteran. USMC. October 1944 through November 1946.
- Served in the Philippine Islands of Leyte, Cebu and Mindanao and recalled to active duty during the Korean Crisis from March 1951 to August 1952.
- Educator (Ret.).

"I do realize the urgency of the POW/MIA Issue. From a personal standpoint, I have no one close to me who is directly involved, with the exception of a friend who was a POW in Germany for a long time.

"Since I am a veteran with dangerous duty in the Philippine Islands before the end of the war, I am fully aware of the conditions under which any POW/MIA lives.

"The current POW/MIA condition still exists as a strange but pertinent predicament. I am retired now. Even though I am a veteran, I cannot commit myself to specific answers.

"Of course, I am aware of the awkward and sad situations of our POW/MIAs. Of course, I want answers from Vietnam. I only hope and pray that the government will solve our problem."

Don Weese:
- State Representative, Oklahoma.
- Vietnam Veteran. B Troop, 1st Squadron, 1st Armord Cavalary Regiment, October 1966 to August 1968.
- Two Purple Hearts, Vietnam Service Medal with four Bronze Stars, Combat Infantryman Badge, Vietnam Campaign Ribbon, Vietnam Gallantry Cross, Unit Badge with Palm.

"I was not in Vietnam at the time of the U.S. withdrawal, having completed my tour and returned home in 1968, well before the withdrawal of troops in the 1970s.

"Any comments I might have are based on my individual belief and opinion and totally without specific knowledge or fact. With that caveat, however . . . .

"I am certain that due to the pressure and haste that was present during the period of withdrawal that confusion, misinformation and periods of chaos or near chaos existed. Operating under those conditions would at least open the possibility that some individuals or groups of individuals could have unknowingly been left behind.

"I also know from my own combat experience that when U.S. Troops were isolated, pinned down or at risk of being killed or captured, no effort was spared to reach and rescue those troops. I personally participated in a number of rescue missions in an area near the border of Laos where I was assigned during my tour of duty in Vietnam in 1967 and 1968.

"If any U.S. personnel were left behind unwillingly, I doubt they are still alive. Once they were discovered or captured they were most probably executed or killed on the spot.

"As I indicated to some degree in my response to question #1, I believe our government should pursue every avenue to identify and account for their presence. Further, we should continue all efforts to identify and account for all those who remain classified as missing in action.

"My thoughts over the past 20 years concerning these questions have not changed.

"Again, the foregoing comments are based solely on my own personal experiences, beliefs and opinions."

Eugene Rockholt:

- Retired-32 years, one month, 19 days, Army; Army Air Corps; U.S. Navy; U.S. Army (16 years in the Special Forces.)
- Two Silver Stars, three Bronze Stars, two Bronze Star Merit, seven Purple Hearts, Meritorious Service Medal, Air Medal, Army Commendation Medal, Air Force Commendation Medal, two Combat Infantry Badges, Master Parachutist Badge (three Countries/U.S., China, Vietnam), Vietnamese Cross of Gallantry: Eighteen Major Campaign Stars (WWII-Korea-Lebanon '58, Vietnam five times.)

"I am convinced that American Servicemen were deliberately and knowingly left behind and declared 'dead' by the powers that be. In my opinion, Dwight D. Eisenhower was the primary force that established the precedent. I am reading, *Kiss The Boys Good-By*.

"I am a member of the Special Forces Association and we have been very active in insisting on accountability of POW/MIAs for years. I am acquainted with 'Bo' Gritz, LTC, Retired from Special Forces, who has been **very** active in the attempt to prove that POW/MIAs were left alive in Vietnam and Laos.

"I think that there is ample evidence in official government files to prove this issue. It only remains that enough pressure be continued to be applied to appropriate officials (Sen. Kerry et. al.) to bring the truth to light.

"No normalization with Vietnam should ever be accorded without complete accounting for our people known to have been in their control."

Jim Weaver:

- WWII Veteran, Normandy Invasion through France, Belguim, Holland and Germany with 38th Armored Infantry Bn. 3rd Army at 17 years of age.
- Korean Veteran. Sergeant, Scout, 1st Marines at Inchon and Chosin Resevoir, hand-to-hand combat, outnumbered 185 to one at 45 degrees below zero.
- Twelve years with Army and Marines.

"Yes, I do think we knowingly left POW/MIAs in Southeast Asia when our troops pulled out in 1973.

"Also, I think some of them are still alive. Our government should have gotten them out at the time of the withdrawal.

"As far as what to do right now, I think our government should go get them. There has been no change in the way I think about Vietnam in the past 20 years."

Bill Weidner:

- VFW State Service Officer with three years, eight months active duty and seven years in Air National Guard, 138th CES.

- Three Air Medals, one Air Force Commendation Medal, Vietnam Service as Crash Fire Fighter/Air Rescue.

"At the time of our troop withdrawal, I didn't think we left anyone over there, now I do.

"I believe some of our people are still alive over there today.

"At the time of our troop withdrawal, our government should not have been so hasty and quick to trust the North Vietnamese.

"As far as right now is concerned, I think the government should quit dragging its feet and quit hiding the facts and just do whatever it takes to admit and correct what has or hasn't been done previously.

"Like most people, I believed what the public was told at first, but now I don't believe what is being said or denied. In the last five years, there seems to be too much evidence in bits and pieces surfacing that leads me to believe our government has made a **big mistake** and tried to cover it up."

Vince Maddex:
- WWI Combat Veteran.
- Fourth Division, 58th Infantry, "L" Company.
- France, Holland, Belgium and Germany.

"I don't know much about those other wars, I didn't fight in them. I always hate to hear people talk about all their fighting when they didn't do any. Our outfit did its share. We used to march all night and then attack at daylight. We did everything on foot back in those days, you know.

"As far as the Vietnam War is concerned, I am like most people who only had the newspapers, TV and the government to tell us what was going on.

"They said back in 1973 that all our American POW/MIAs were dead. I have always found that to be strange since Americans keep surfacing every year or so even though the government said they were all dead.

"I do think some of those POWs could still be alive. We never should have stopped bombing and fighting until they were all accounted for. I had a great Nephew in the Gulf War and that's the way Gen. Powell did it in that war. He demanded a full accounting of our POW/MIAs or we'd keep on fighting until we got them all back. The government did not do that in the Vietnam War. So, we should never lift the embargo until Americans are accounted for and we are satisfied.

"The Vietnamese were our enemies. Why should we believe them back then or right now? We should load up and go get our boys out. We have the right stuff to do it too.

"I still think just like I did 20 years ago about Vietnam. We left some there, we shouldn't have quit fighting until they were accounted for and we should go back and get the ones that are left."

Robert Scott:
- Vietnam Combat Veteran. Scout, Squad Leader.
- Purple Heart, Bronze Star, Combat Infantry Badge.

"Yes, I think we left quite a few of them over there. I think some of them are still alive. If a man has the will to live, he'll try it.

"We had the power to go back in there and bomb them with B-52s. We should have negotiated at that time with North Vietnam and made it clear we wanted a full accounting for our missing troops or we'd bomb them until they complied.

"I think the North Vietnamese are still lying about it. I think we should still negotiate hard with them. You're just giving in to what they want by lifting the embargo and trading with them. These were our enemies and still are until they tell the truth about our POW/MIAs.

"We used to have to fight in Cambodia and I lost some men in there and I've always wondered if their loved ones got the military benefits due them since we were 'supposedly' not fighting in there. I've always wondered what would have happened if I had been captured or killed while over in Cambodia fighting.

"We really thought we were making America proud by fighting and dying over there, but now it doesn't seem that they were proud of us at all. At least they never showed it. I wonder if soldiers of other wars ever felt they risked their lives for nothing? It's sad if they do."

Captain Eugene B. "Red" McDaniel:
- USAF Pilot, Retired.
- POW in North Vietnam over six years.
- The Navy Cross, two Silver Stars, The Legion of Merit with Combat "V", the Distinguished Flying Cross, three Bronze Stars with Combat "V", and two Purple Hearts as North Vietnamese POW.
- Author: *Scars and Stripes.*

"Yes! We left Americans in Southeast Asia when our troops withdrew in 1973. Three former Secretaries of Defense, Laird, Richardson and Schlensgen, testified before Select Committee, 352 in Laos, 244 in Vietnam.

"Are any still alive? There are 135 discrepancies in Vietnam plus those in Laos that are not yet accounted for.

"Back then, our government should have told the truth, (we had no leverage to lose) rather than lie to the families.

"Now, they should make a serious effort to return the live POWs or remains of those left in Southeast Asia and Korea, plus those taken from Vietnam to Russia.

"I was a POW for over six and a half years in Hanoi and it looks like they could have ended the war and gotten us all out long before they did. I learned just 10 years ago that we left some behind and I still believe it."

Douglass W. Penny:

- Vietnam Veteran.
- Combat Engineer Sgt. 101st Airborne Infantry, U.S. Army.
- Purple Heart, Presidential Unit Citation, Vietnam Gallantry Medal, Parachute Badge.
- Six years in the service of America.

"I think there are POW/MIAs still in Vietnam and Laos.

"We should go get them out. Vietnam should at least be accountable for the remains of all the Americans who we know for a fact are being held.

"Government officials should never lift sanctions against Vietnam until America is fully satisfied. This means all live POW/MIAs and remains of American POW/MIAs."

Don Nickles:

- U.S. Senator.

"Concerning the return of American POW/MIAs who may still be in captivity in Southeast Asia, I believe we must do everything within our power to secure an accounting of all 2,264 Amerians who are still listed as missing in action as a result of the war in Vietnam.

"It is imperative that every American service member know that when a person is lost defending his or her country, the United States will not rest until their family is cared for and an exact accounting is obtained of his or her whereabouts.

"We cannot rest knowing there is a chance that an American is being held captive under the type of conditions our servicemen were held in North Vietnam during the war. For that reason, we must continue to assume that some Americans are still alive. Then, we should work to our utmost to determine their fate and secure their return.

"The possibility of live POWs and reports in the press about possible leads are matters of great concern to me. I have been briefed on the matter thoroughly by the Office of the Seceretary of Defense and have been in contact with the Justice Department, the Department of State, and the Defense Intelligence Agency. According to the DOS's Office of International Security Affairs there are 39 full-time investigators working on reports on the POW/MIA situation.

"It is imperative that each bit of information be investigated in detail and each country involved in this issue cooperate to bring the POW/MIAs home. The administration has and will continue to respond to the request of any congressmen. I have been pledged the full cooperation of any investigation needed.

"Please be assured I am firmly committed to do all I can to secure the release of any American POWs still held in Southeast Asia and to obtain the return of any remains for proper identification."

Charles C. Zotter:

- Vietnam Veteran. USMC. 1968-1970. HQ 1-233rd Air Defense Artillery.
- Vietnamese Cross of Gallantry, Unit Citation with Palm Leaf.
- Combat Action Ribbon, Vietnam Service Medal with two Bronze Stars, Vietnam Campaign Medal, Army Commendation Medal, Army Achievement Medal, Arkansas Commendation Medal.
- Bachelor of Arts Degree with High Honors at Ark. Tech Univ.
- Working on Masters Thesis.

"As with all Vietnam veterans, with the passing years the recollections have faded as we get on with our lives. It is not very often that my Vietnam experience comes to mind anymore. Like the other veterans, they are filled with painful memories. I am still not sure if it is the closeness to my fellow Marines, the loss of friends through death, or the manner in which we were treated upon returning home, but to this day I get very sad when I try to recall the years 1969-1970. However, I will attempt to answer the questions to the best of my ability and perhaps expound upon them somewhat.

"Did we knowingly leave prisoners in Southeast Asia when our forces left? As far as I am concerned the answer is yes. Why our government did not force the issue I am not sure. I suppose they were a little embarrassed since Vietnam was the first war we had lost since the War of 1812. Furthermore, the war was very political and I imagine the politicians wished to sweep it under the rug as soon as possible.

"I believe the POWs in Vietnam were abandoned by our politicians. Perhaps they hoped they would die off and everyone would simply forget. But, Americans do not forget. The North Vietnamese took prisoners, did not adhere to the Geneva Convention, and now, they are haunted by concerned Americans who constantly irritate them about our POWs. We may never get them back, or their remains, but the next country we go to war with will have learned the lesson that they had better account for our POWs, because even if politicians don't care, the American people do.

"Are some of these prisoners still alive? Yes! I am still alive, so there is no reason why they are not. The North Vietnamese do not wish to release them because they will relay the atrocities committed upon them. They are probably being used in force labor camps or kept in isolation somewhere. If they are not alive, that means that the North Vietnamese killed them, and that makes them guilty of war crimes. (Why did we spend so much time and effort trying the German war criminals and not even make an attempt to bring the North Vietnamese to justice?)

"What the government should have done at the time is they should have commenced with saturation bombing of Hanoi 24 hours a day around the clock until every POW was accounted for. As far as the world opinion is concerned, since when have our politicians cared about world opinion? They have made us the laughing stock of the world and have practically rewarded the rest of the world for laughing at us.

"But, realistically, there is nothing they can do. America is tied up in world economy. We have signed so many treaties and agreements, our trade and commerce is worldwide; we no longer have the option of being isolationists. Early in our history our founding fathers warned of entangling alliance and no sooner did the words fall out of their mouths until we entered into an alliance with France during the American Revolution. The framers of the Constitution were of the moneyed class. They were educated and owned businesses and property. They considered the common man 'too stupid' to make decisions and that is why there were property qualifications in order to vote.

"Yes, we have come a long way since then—but not far enough.

Larry D. Forrester:
• Manufacturer's Representative.

"My interest in the POW/MIA Issue derives from the fact that my brother, Lt. Ron W. Forrester, has been Missing-in-Action since December 27, 1972.

"I'm not sure we knowingly left prisoners. Some experts involved in the issue in the time frame say we did. Certainly, we failed to press Vietnam for an accounting of the 70 known discrepancy cases.

"Seventy men were known to have been on the ground alive or alive in North Vietnam Prison Camps, yet, at the war's conclusion, we failed to keep the issue alive. This is abominable. Of course, we need to resolve as many MIA cases as soon as possible.

"Only Vietnam knows. They certainly know more than they've admitted thus far. This is a documented fact.

"Our government should have given priority status to the issue.

"Normalization of relations with Vietnam should not take place until we're convinced they have done all they can do.

"Recent revelations from WWII and the Korean War make me skeptical of our government and their commitment to the issue.

"Responding to a recent newspaper article, I wrote the following editorial:

"'Dear Editor;

Your article entitled 'To Laos and Back' was wrought with misguided patriotism. Despite Dr. Kissinger's denials, he certainly knew, as the facts are well-documented, that all POWs, known to have been alive while in captivity of the enemy, were not returned nor was a case of doublespeak. He says, 'Other prisoners could have been held but we didn't have proof.' Please! That sounds like, (I don't know and I don't want to know.)

"The sacrifices of the gallant fighting men who were placed in harm's way demand that we account for their fate, even if we can only confirm that they belong to God. As has been proven by the testimonies of diverse defectors, the North Vietnamese hold many answers. The Nixon government never shouted the questions loud enough for them to be heard.

"Yes! The Politics of the Vietnam era were troubled, and true, the senators (all of whom are not anti-war liberals) who push for the truth are stepping back into the quagmire. But, sir, the families of the missing have been bogged down in that quagmire since the chaplain showed up on the doorstep with the awful news that their loved one was missing.

"Give Senator Kerry his due. The Senate Select Committee on POW/MIA Affairs hearings have been conducted with the utmost probity. Certainly, questions are being asked that **should have been asked in 1973,** regardless of the political atmosphere of the period, or despite of political consequences.

"Please write what you write as if your son were missing in action! Write in favor of an accounting, rather than lambasting those who seek to supply the balm of badly-needed answers."

Larry D. Forrester

Leslie L. Brown:
- POW WWII. "E" Btry. 60th C.A.C. (AA) Btry "Way 12" mortors.
- 1,201 days as a POW; Five and a half years in service.
- Baatan and Battle of Corregidor.
- Presidential Unit Citations, Purple Heart, POW Medal, Oklahoma Cross of Valor, American Defense with Foreign Service Clasp, Asiatic Pacific Medal with two Stars, Victory Medal, Philippine Defense Medal, seven overseas bars and enough memories to last a lifetime.

"Yes, I think the government left some of our POW/MIAs when the American troops withdrew from Southeast Asia.

"I sure think it's possible that there are some still alive today.

"Back then, at the time of the withdrawal, the government should have been more forceful and kept our word on the agreement on helping POWs.

"As far as right now is concerned, obviously the government should make sure none are held against their will.

"How my thoughts have changed over the past 20 years? I don't think we should have been there in the first place. The French were kicked out, as they should have been. Their leader asked Truman for help to get the French out at the end of WWII.

"We gave up the Philippines in 1946. The French should have done the same thing. They had earned their freedom fighting the Japanese. Our standing would have been much greater today and some 50,000 young men would be alive today.

"Our Foreign Policy is bad. The Shaw of Iran, Somozon in Nicaraqua, Batista in Cuba, Marcos in the Philippines and we almost lost Korea. You can't dictate other peoples' lives."

Cletys Nordin:
- POW Korean War from December 31, 1950 until August 23, 1953.
- K Company, 19th Regt. 24th Inf. Division.

"It is my opinion that we probably didn't leave any Americans in Southeast Asia *knowingly*.

"Also, it seems very doubtful that any would still be alive today.

"The government should have searched more back then, and continue to search today.

"My thoughts haven't changed about Vietnam at all in the past 20 years. I was a POW and I know what our boys had to go through. We should continue to search for them and never give up.

"On New Year's Day, 1951, I and 1,000 other American POWs began the Death March. We walked every night for seven weeks, the length of North Korea, from the 38th Parallel, all the way up the the Yalu River, bordering China. That winter, 1,400 of the 3,000 prisoners died from starvation, sickness and bad treatment.

"We should continue to search for our POWs and never give up."

Glenn E. Peterson:
- POW WWII, U.S. Army, Co. H, 180th Inf, 45th Div.
- Four and a half years in the military.
- POW Medal, Combat Infantry Badge, American Defense Medal, European Defense Medal, two Battle Stars, Oklahoma Cross of Valor.

"We probably left Americans in Southeast Asia but I don't think we knowingly did.

"I do not believe that there are any Americans still alive in Vietnam, Laos or Cambodia.

"My thoughts on Vietnam and these questions haven't changed any in the past 20 years."

Raymond W. Brumbach:

- POW Korean War Veteran.
- Second Inf. Division.
- POW three times, escaped three times, three Purple Hearts, Silver Star, Bronze Star, POW Medal, four Battle Stars.

"My story appeared in the March issue of *The American Legion* magazine.

"I was a POW, I got out. I only wish all Americans who have been held in captivity could have gotten out.

"In Korea, I was wounded three times, captured three times, escaped three times, I have three children, so I guess three is my lucky, or unlucky number.

"I remember when the 2nd Infantry Division was overrun by the Chinese, they lined up 15 American Prisoners and killed every third one. I was one of those 15 prisoners who was lined up. That is just one of the three's in my life.

"Personally, I don't know if the government intentionally left behind Amerian POW/MIAs. Not that they didn't, but I don't know if they did.

"I don't believe there are any Americans alive that were POW/MIAs back then.

"At the time of the withdrawal in 1973, the government should have done more research on POW/MIAs.

"As far as now goes, they should keep searching.

"Off and on at different times, my thoughts have changed about Vietnam and the POW/MIAs during the past 20 years . . . but, they should keep searching."

Oscar S. Sparks:

- POW WWII, Germany, December 25, 1944 to May 1, 1945.
- Army Air Corps, Combat Fighter Bombers, 314th F.S. 432th F.G., 12th A.C.
- Distinguished Flying Cross, nine Air Medals, two Purple Hearts, POW Medal, Various Unit Citations.

"World War II started for me in May 1944, flying P-40 Fighter Bombers. We fought at Cercola, Pignatero and Anzio. Then, we got some P-47s and went on into France. Near Kaiserlautern, Germany, I was shot down and had to parachute out. I was captured on Christmas Day 1944, moved to many prison camps over Germany and was at last liberated when the Russians overran our POW Camp at the end of April, 1945.

"Yes, I do believe the government left some of our people in Southeast Asia at the time of withdrawal.

"I do think some of them are still alive but I don't think we'll ever see them.

"We should have clearcut won the War. We had the capabilities but not the political backing (as in Korea).

"Today, we should treat Vietnam as if they didn't exist.

"No! My thoughts have not mellowed about Vietnam over the past 20 years. And . . . I would treat Japan as if they had the plague."

Leif Robert Olson:
- WW II. 12 years in Service. U.S. Army & U.S. Air Force.
- Pilot, Bombadier, Navigator, Intelligence, Radio Operator, Parachute Rigger, Gunnery Observer.
- Service Medals, Presidential Citations, Unit Citations.
- Awarded Wartime Service Disability for duty performed.

"Yes, we did knowingly leave prisoners in Southeast Asia when our forces left the field of action. We also have left prisoners in other wars or engagements in the past century. Remember the more than 8,000 still unaccounted for during the Korean War.

"It is possible that there are some living prisoners from the Vietnam War in Southeast Asia. There is a possibility some prisoners moved to other continent areas and are still alive. More likely than not, they are now absorbed into the local existence of the country they were isolated to.

"At the time of the Vietnam War, our government should have made an intense effort to free those imprisoned veterans. If we can go to war over a few barrels of oil, our service persons deserve equal compassion and backup with arms as necessary.

"Now, the government should publish the truth and names of those who officially gave the orders to leave our service personnel at the mercy of the enemy government."

Barney Oldfield:
- USAF (Ret.): Founder & Secretary of Foundation of the Americas for the Handicapped; Luftwaffe/U.S. Air Force International Friendship Foundation; Founder & Treasurer, Radio & TV News Directors Foundation; Founder, Aviation/Space Writers Foundation; Trustee, U.S. Air Force Museum Foundation, Univ. of Nebraska Film Society; Radio & TV News Association of Southern California, Radio & TV News Directors Assn.
- Overseas Press Club of America, Greater Los Angeles Press Club, Armed Forces Broadcasters Assn.; American Film Institute; sixth winner in 43 years of the Radio & TV News Directors Assn.; Distinguished Service Award; Dubbed "King of the Press Agents" by Charles Kuralt on CBS WHO's WHO; Newsletter, PR REPORTER, designation as "Best Speech Writer;" 1983 Selection as Distinguished Nebraskalander of the Year; Honorary Degree, Doctor of Letters, University of Nebraska; VFW Distinguished Citizen, 1992.

"I have absolutely no competence to judge in this matter as I retired, hung up the uniform in September 1962, and ran off to Copacabana Beach to watch the Cuban Missile Crisis from the underside—and Vietnam was one I missed. Considering what an awful legacy it has been for those who knew it, or like our new leader, did everything possible to keep from knowing it, I'm not sorry to have been denied it.

"For 30 years, three months and 28 days, I went everywhere the bells rang—33 countries in all, War, Peace and Cold War (NATO).

"I can only wish you well in your quest to find answers about America's POW/MIAs, and that I do . . . ."

David Edward Fortune:
- Korean Veteran. POW two years and seven months. Eleven months in hard labor.
- Three times retired, U.S. Civil Service, Army Reserve, Assistant Veterans Affairs Officer, 13 1/2 years active duty, 27 years reserve.
- Retired as a Chief warrant officer, W4.
- Combat Infantry Badge, Good Conduct Medal, Army Commendation, Meritorious Service and the Legion of Merit Medals. Several others including the POW Medal.

"Yes, I believe with all my heart that we knowingly left live prisoners of war behind, not only in Southeast Asia but also in Korea and World War II. For these three wars there are 81,000 Americans not accounted for at wars end.

"Yes, it is my firm belief that once a person makes the big adjustment to the treatment, weather, food and many other conditions, he can exist indefinitely.

"The government should have taken whatever action necessary to achieve a full accounting. During World War II, Americans were buried on British soil and never brought home. They were lost at sea off the coast of France and not recovered and they were taken to Russia to never be heard from again.

"In Korea, Americans were sent to both China and Russia to never be heard from again. I was personally in a group of about 104 Americans that the Chinese were going to keep until a British POW got the attention of a Red Cross person who demanded to see the POW and then made it his business to see that the remainder of us were also exchanged.

"The government should continue to seek a full accounting of all of our people. Every American who fought and died for our country and our beliefs of freedom for all people, deserves the right to at least be buried in a marked cemetery, whether here at home or in a foreign country and his family deserves the right to know the *true* information about their loved ones, 'Lest We Forget.'

"Today, I do not trust our intelligence community or our accountability people as far as one can toss the Statue of Liberty. I think Col. Peck is a National

Hero for what he did in his effort to expose the accountability coverup.

"All of the classified information about our POW/MIAs, except for our foreign agents, should be made public. Let the families of those not accounted for judge whether our government has been honest or not.

"What ever happened to 'We The People?'"

Harrison Sallisbury:

- Harper/Collins.
- International Political Writer.

"I don't think we left any prisoners behind—not knowingly. There may have been a handful of special cases of one sort or another. But these were inadvertent.

"None of these prisoners (if there were any) are still alive.

"The government should have thoroughly investigated these prisoners at the time. There is nothing it can do now. My thoughts have not changed over the years."

William L. Culver:

- Lt. Col. USAF (Ret.).
- One hundred-fifty combat missions during Vietnam War.

"It is important that we give credit to the many brave men who have fought to protect the principles on which our country is founded.

"We need to continue the cycle of educating our children in the values that are worth defending with life and blood, and teach them the importance of carefully choosing what, where, and when we will fight. There is nothing like hearing it from the lips of the men who have 'been there.'

"I don't have any 'special' knowledge or qualifications that would make a difference in the POW/MIA Issue. I have never met anyone who professed to have any knowledge about POWs left behind in Southeast Asia.

"I had a friend who served on the team that went back in to recover some of the remains (fatalities, not POWs) in the late 1980s. I only talked to him twice and he could shed no light on the subject that I hadn't already heard in the media.

"However, I never gave up hoping that a POW might turn up. For the most part, the men I have served with have been honest, upright, and forthright who would not knowingly participate in or condone a cover-up.

"This feeling of confidence in our leadership has increased significantly in the past 20 years. I certainly did not have this same confidence when I left Vietnam."

Michael Lee Lanning:
- 2/3 199th Light Infantry Bde. 1969-1970.
- Twenty years in service.
- Bronze Star with Valor, two Oak Leaf Clusters Defense Meritorious Service Medal with Oak Leaf Cluster Air Medal, Army Commendation Medal, Combat infantryman's Badge, Senior Parachutist.
- Served in Infantry, Airborne, Ranger and Armor.

"Did we knowingly leave prisoners in Southeast Asia when our forces left is not clear. The *we* as in the *we* of the 2.5 million servicemen and women who served with honor in Vietnam certainly did not knowingly leave any of our comrades behind.

"If it is *we,* as in Henry Kissinger and friends, then this is a different question. As a professional soldier with more than 20 years of service and a half-dozen books to my credit published about the war, I can only answer for *we* that served, and *we* knowingly left no one behind.

"Are some of these prisoners still alive? There are anywhere from one-half to a dozen American deserters known to be living in Vietnam today. As for Americans being held against their will, there is no proof that any remain. Anyone seriously looking at this question must ask themselves, 'What is in it for the Vietnamese?' The answer is that there is nothing to their advantage to still have live prisoners and I do not think that they do so. As for remains, and additional information on their deaths, that is a different matter.

"What should the government have done at the time? The government was never able to establish a mission for the war itself, much less POW issues. If one must point a finger and establish blame, then the entire country is responsible. The people of the United States wanted the war to end regardless of the cost.

"Two thousand-plus MIAs, especially when most were professional, career military men, seemed like a cheap price to politicians wanting to ensure their re-electability and to the anti-war, anti-military forces that wanted peace at any price.

"What should the government do now? They should continue to deny diplomatic recognition and continue trade restrictions until Vietnam reveals all available (whatever that is) information in regard to MIAs. (Many) American businessmen care not about the war, the warriors or the MIAs. All they want to do is open another profitable market for their wares. They think with their pocketbooks rather than their hearts or heads.

"How have my thoughts about these questions changed over the past 20 years? Obviously, there has been a great deal of information, and some evidence, that MIAs may have been left behind. If this is true, it is about the only issue that would make this old soldier pick up his ruck sack, shoulder a M-16 and be ready to return to Vietnam to complete what we left unfinished.

"Another thought about the POW/MIA issue comes to mind. It seems that many individuals and groups use the POW/MIA issue as a means to further their own causes and ambitions with little real concern for, or understanding about, the MIAs and their families."

William T. Bennett:
• General Secretary.
  National Vietnam Veterans Coalition, Washington, D.C.

"These responses represent my (present) personal view. Did we knowingly leave prisoners in Southeast Asia when our forces left? Yes. Beneath the semantic subterfuges of the executive summary of the Select Senate Committee on POW/MIA Final Report, the point is made irrefutably. Numerous lists had been compiled of known and suspected POWs (e.g. the categories, the CINCPAC list of between 350 and 450, a DIA list of 130, the WSAG estimate of 40 POWs in Laos, etc.) who did not return.

"Given due regard to the 'semantic subterfuge,' it is possible that no one could pinpoint with any degree of precision precisely who was held prisoner and where.

"The question further presupposes that the U.S. government had an option in the matter. I think not. Henry Kissinger, in his senate testimony, could almost, but not quite, bring himself to admit the following: because of the revulsion against the war, by 1973 the government was stripped of all negotiating tools—force was not an option, due to Cooper-Church and other legislative crippler amendments; nor could the POWs be ransomed out, because Congress would not approve an aid package envisioned in President Nixon's secret letter.

"Are some of the prisoners still alive? Possibly, probably. The Select Senate Committee investigators entrusted with review of the POW intelligence have offered estimates as high as 850. But there is apparently little that is regarded by even Senator Bob Smith as definitive since 1989.

"What should the government have done at the time? Just about anything other than what it did do. It should have publicly admitted the problem instead of employing semantically misleading terminology, such as 'no current information' that there are POWs alive in SEA; it should have reclassified MIAs as POWs in accordance with the wishes of the service secretaries instead of the other way around; it should not have commissioned public speeches by the likes of William Clements and Chappie James which blasted the activists on the issue. It should have continued intelligence, and even increased intelligence priorities instead of downgrading them almost to the point of zero.

"What should the government do now? Continue the trade embargo. Upgrade the intelligence priorities, but this time start by cleaning house of the professional debunkers at the Defense Intelligence Agency.

"How have my thoughts about these questions changed over the past 20 years? They are constantly in a state of flux. This answer is different, for example, than the one I would have given a week ago, because in the interval, I have had the opportunity to review various Select Senate Committee documents on file at the National Archives, which I have referenced in my first answer."

William L. (Bert) McCollum:
- Combat Infantry Badge.
- Bronze Star. Bronze Arrowhead Asiatic-Pacific Campaign Ribbon, Philippine Liberation Ribbon with one Bronze Star, Good Conduct Medal, Army of Occupation Ribbon, Japan Victory Ribbon, Three Overseas Service Bars.

"I served four years in the Pacific during World War II. Then I also spent 13 months and seven years in Korea with the 6th Infantry Division.

"I believe that the U.S. government knowingly left prisoners behind when our troops pulled out of Vietnam. Under combat conditions sometimes some of that cannot be helped, especially the kind of war we were requiring our troops to fight over there. That was a very hard fight for our men.

"I doubt any might still be alive after all this time, considering the treatment the Vietnamese dished out to our POWs.

"I believe they actually tried to get our POWs out, but I don't think they did enough for our MIAs.

"We should not seek normal relations with Vietnam until they are honest about our MIAs.

"I have not changed my thought about the war in Vietnam, except for the fact that now I realize more than ever that the American soldiers did everything that was demanded of them just like they did when I was fighting in the Pacific during WWII. They did what they were told. They deserve much more recognition and respect."

William S. (Bill) Vardeman:
- U.S. Navy 1940-1945. Chief Aviator Radio Man and enlisted pilot in Okinawa.
- U.S. Air Force 1947-1969.
- 121st Fighter Wing, Ohio National Guard, Korea War Veteran.
- Retired after 22 years in service as Major.

"Yes, our government did leave prisoners behind in Southeast Asia when our forces left in 1973.

"I still believe some of those prisoners may be alive, however, some of them may have asked to stay by now. We should have tried to get them before the war ended. We should always keep trying to get them out.

"My thoughts about Vietnam have not changed over the past 20 years.

William Brocker:
- U.S. Marines, 17-years old.
- 0311 Infantry.
- In the Vietnam War from February 1971 to January 3, 1973.

"When the POWs came out of North Vietnam I could not believe how few there were. My Dad had been a bombardier in WWII. More than once I had heard him say that air crews that fell into Russian hands were never heard from again. Dad seemed to think the government wrote them off. As it turns out, he was correct.

"I cannot help but believe that the U.S. government, in their lust to placate the hippies, yuppies, and future presidents, wrote our men off as before. Nixon purchased our way out of Vietnam, and the North Vietnam Army held onto POWs as security. We didn't keep our part and Uncle Ho didn't keep his part.

"All this is a bit retrospective. When Bush laid out the 'road for normal relations,' I believe it sealed the fate of any living American in Vietnam or Laos. Any evidence of holding POWs after that time would cause Vietnam and Laos to lose face.

"I suspect that before withdrawal, we should have held out in our negotiations for a complete accounting in joint sessions between the North Vietnamese, Viet Cong, South Vietnamese and ourselves.

"While Vietnam was a quagmire, it was a quagmire created by LBJ, Congress and the State Department, formulating the most rigid rules of engagement ever imposed upon a military campaign.

"Like everyone else associated with Vietnam, I want a full accounting. Recognization of Vietnam is fundamentally wrong. If you lie down with dogs, you will generally wind up with fleas.

"Over the past 20 years, my opinion on POW/MIAs has not changed. Rather, each revelation has reinforced my beliefs."

John Reid III:
- Editor, *Delaware County Journal*.
- First Bn. 3rd Marines, Vietnam 1967-1968.
- Fifth Communication Bn. Vietnam 1969-1970.
- Served 25 months in Vietnam.
- Radio-Telephone Operator-Artillery & Naval Forward Observer.
- Participated in 29 Combat Operations as part of Special Landing Force.
- Received Combat Action Ribbon. Presidential Unit Citation.
- Republic of Vietnam Unit Awards.

"In my opinion, the United States did not knowingly or unknowingly leave behind POWs and none were kept by the North Vietnamese or Viet Cong after the return of POWs in 1972.

"No evidence exists of POWs being kept and no military or political purpose would have been served by keeping them. A full accounting of the deaths of those listed as MIAs should be obtained from whatever source possible."

Oliver North:
- USMC (Ret.).
- Twenty-two years of service.
- Vietnam Veteran serving 13 months in combat.
- Wounded five times and awarded two Purple Hearts, the Silver
  Star, the Bronze Star with V for Valor, three Navy Commendations
  Medals, and Vietnam Campaign Medals.

"To help families of the missing cope with the falsehoods, anxiety, and sometimes seeming intransigence of their own government, a group of POW/MIA wives organized to support one another and to the extent they could, help their men in bondage.

"Initially headed by Sybil Stockdale, the wife of Navy flyer James Stockdale who was a POW, the group eventually incorporated as a nonprofit foundation in 1970. Today, the National League of Families of American Prisoners and Missing in Southeast Asia has over 3,500 members nationwide.

"These brave women actively campaigned to make the world aware of the brutal treatment their men were receiving long before Operation Homecoming. After the releases in 1973, those who did come home confirmed that their treatment improved as a consequence of the League's work.

"But nearly 2,300 men remained unaccounted for, and because progress in finding remains and resolving reports is so painstakingly slow, every organization involved, the League of Families and the U.S. government included, has been subjected to criticism.

"Conspiracy theories, 'cover-up' stories, and accusations abound. Sadly, none of this has helped advance the resolution of what has happened to missing Americans.

"Lt. Col. Jack Donovan, heading the U.S. Task Force-Full Accounting Team of Army, Air Force, Navy and Marine experts universally, said they did not believe that the Hanoi government was holding any live Americans, although they willingly admitted that they could not prove it and that it was entirely possible that in the hitherlands, or in Laos, some Americans could be held by 'warlords' outside the control of the government."

When Lt. Col. North returned from a recent trip to North Vietnam and after he had read some of the reports to Congress on the effectiveness of the Task Force, he drew some very interesting conclusions:

- The cooperation of the Vietnamese government with our effort to locate, recover and identify American remains has slowly but steadily improved since it began with a visit in 1982 by Deputy Assistant Secretary of Defense Richard Armitage who had started the ball rolling.

- The average Vietnamese is more than a little baffled about the American focus on this issue. Their puzzlement is the consequence of the dramatic differences between their culture and ours, and one very stark fact: The people of Vietnam still cannot account for more than 330,000 of their own sons and daughters lost, on both sides, in the war between 1960-1975.

- For those who trudged through the mountainous, triple-canopied jungle, such a number is not surprising. But, more astonishing is that the number of Americans missing or unaccounted for is as low as it is.

"Much of Vietnam's lush foliage is so dense that entering it is like being devoured by nature. Given the severity of much of the terrain, the humid tropical climate, the animals of the wild, and the sparse population outside the country's towns and cities, it is a tribute to American bravery and persistence that the number isn't much higher.

"In all, counting the confirmed dead and MIAs, the United States lost more than 60,000 of its sons and daughters in Southeast Asia. Because battlefield search and rescue technology had significantly improved, the medevac capabilities had advanced, it was possible to retrieve the bodies of more than 95 percent of all those who fell in Vietnam.

"This far surpasses the tally for other modern conflicts. Nearly three times as many Americans never returned from Korea and 78,794 of those who served in WWII remain unaccounted for. Those numbers from other wars, of course, do nothing to assuage the lingering pain, sadness, emptiness, and anger felt by those who sent a loved one off to war who never returned.

"But even though those who served in Vietnam did a better job of returning the remains of our fallen comrades-in-arms than in prior wars, the issue has ignited stronger passions in Vietnam than any other modern war. Why?

"In the nearly two decades since the end of the war, the POWs and MIAs have come to symbolize American sentiment about the Vietnam war. The black POW/MIA banner with its white silhouette of an American POW in a barbed-wire enclosure and a guard tower is now commonplace in schools, churches, parades, and civic functions across America.

"It is the smaller version of this logo, worn as a patch, that one sees on so many of the camouflage-clad vets on America's city streets. The kind of deep regard Americans display toward our POWs and MIAs reflects a preexisting emotional attachment to this issue. Why does this issue captivate us as it does?

"It may well be that for many Americans, veterans and others, the POWs/MIAs have become the one issue that unites us all about the war. By the late 1960s, the turmoil and confusion over American involvement in Vietnam led to a national condition of ambivalence.

"When those who served did not come home as they had fought—in squads, platoons, companies, and battalions, but alone, one-by-one, occasionally harassed, sometimes scorned, but mostly unnoticed—the issue of Vietnam remained unsettled. The only ones who came home to a heroes' welcome were the POWs who returned together, as a group.

"General Vessey's formula, developed by an aging warrior but grounded in the solid Judeo-Christian teaching about clothing the naked and feeding the hungry, has provided us with an opportunity to complete the mission we failed to finish as a nation.

"By actively engaging in providing help, directly from one people to another, outside the framework of government, Vietnam, whether alive of dead, well or maimed, home or not."

Carol Hrdlicka
- Wife of POW left in Southeast Asia
- U.S. Air Force

"Why wasn't Col. David Hrdlicka ever released from Laos? On May 18, 1965, Col. David Hrdlicka was the lead pilot of a F-105 mission when he was hit by ground fire and his aircraft caught fire. He ejected and parachuted into a valley near a village in the Sam Neua area of Laos.

"His wingman saw him land and watched helplessly as native people rolled up his parachute and led him away. A helicopter landed in a nearby village a short time later and the pilot was told that the downed airman had been turned over to Pathet Lao troops.

"On July 22, 1966, the story of David Hrdlicka's capture was published in *Ouan Nhan Dan,* a North Vietnamese newspaper. A few days later, a personal letter purportedly written by David, was broadcast both in Southeast Asia and by Radio Peking.

"One month later in Moscow, *Pravda* published a photograph of David Hrdlicka. The Defense Intelligence Agency also had a post-capture photograph album of POWs and under David's photo, The DIA typed,

"David Louis Hrdlicka," so we may safely assume that he has been positively identified to the satisfaction of our own experts.

"The extensive cave complex in the Sam Neua area is carved out of solid rock. The Pathet Lao headquarters survived massive bombing because the caves were impervious to attack. It is believed that many of the prisoners captured by the Pathet Lao were incarcerated deep in these caves both during and after the war.

"*Pravda* correspondent, Ivan Shchedrov, interviewed David Hrdlicka in May of 1969. He had survived for four years. The Pathet Lao has never turned over one single POW and they are known to have had many.

"A White House memorandum from the Situation Room to Henry Kissinger on June 9, 1973 stated, 'The Pathet Lao's chief representative in Vientiane on June 8 accepted a personal letter from Mrs. Emmet Kay to her husband . . . but told our Embassy officer that further information on two other acknowledged POWs (David Hrdlicka and Eugene De Bruin) must await the formation of a new coalition government in Laos.'

"Emmet Kay was ultimately released but Hrdlicka and De Bruin were not. DPMO has records of David Hrdlicka being seen alive in Laos as late as June, 1989.

"What happened to the men who were known to be alive in captivity? Why is it the government is only asking for bodies? What about the known, documented POWs?"

The following is Mrs. Hrdlicka's reponses to several questions:

Did we knowingly leave prisoners in Southeast Asia when our forces left? "Yes, there are many documents that back this statement, not to mention the testimony given before the Senate Select Committee by former Secretaries of Defense and other high-ranking officials."

Are some of these prisoners still alive? "Yes, there are at this time 48 authenticator codes picked up by satellite imagery from Southeast Asia—some as late as 1992. There were two men who put there authenticator codes down six times in 20 years but no one answered these distress signals. Authenticator codes are four-digit numbers assigned to pilots to be used only as distress signals and for purpose of identification when captured, imprisoned, etc. There is overwhelming evidence in the form of live-sighting reports as well. I have documents tracking POWs in the 1980s. If there were no men left and no men alive, why were U.S. Government agencies wasting taxpayers' dollars tracking people whom they publicly implied did not exist?"

What should our government have done at the time? "Taken the facts to the floor of Congress and asked for the $4.2 billion in aid promised to the Vietnamese by President Nixon—use this as a bargaining chip—gone to the Laotians and demanded a seperate peace treaty. The Laotians had told the U.S. Government that they had men and would release them *only* if negotiations were held in Vientiane. Our government should have been truthful with the families of the imprisoned or missing men as well as the American people concerning the number of men known to be alive and in captivity—those not returned at Homecoming 1973–instead of withholding the truth and continuing to withhold it to this day.

What should our government do now? "Our government should finally admit the full truth. They should contact the Vietnamese and tell them there will be NO recriminations if they immediately release all remaining living POWs as well as the remains of all who have died in captivity. Being faced with the overwhelming accumulated evidence, the Vietnamese would have to either produce or show full proof that there are no men alive. Only then should the repatriation promised by Richard Nixon be paid."

Have your thoughts about the POW/MIA issue changed over the past 20 or more years? "I have come to realize that our government (which I trusted) has in affect lied to the families and the general public about the men they knowingly abandoned–purposely keeping information from the families instead of including them in the investigation. Had the government been honest years ago, many of these men could have been bought out by family members without any great disgrace to anyone."

John L. (Lepp) Leppelman:
- Thirty-five months in Vietnam.
- 173rd Airborne, Army Riverboats, All-volunteer Rangers, LRRP.
- Bronze Star with "V" device, the Army Commendation Medal, the Air Medal, the Purple Heart, South Vietnam Cross of Gallantry, the Combat Infantryman Badge, Parachute Wings, Vietnam Service Medal with three Bronze Stars and one Silver Star, Valorous Unit Emblem.

"I was back in Vietnam a year ago on a POW search interviewing Ex-CIA and Chinese Agents. It was very interesting and it would take too much room to try to put it down now.

"But, I can tell you that we still have men over there as well as in Russia. Our government has written them off."

Vietnam Veterans of America Chapter 672 Newsletter, Tulsa, OK, Keith Cook, Secretary–Vietnam Veteran

"Our State Chairman of POW/MIA Affairs of America, Bob Stephens, who was a Vietnam Veteran, spent 20 years involved with every issue of POW/MIAs. He was the primary instrument in getting a proclamation entered into the State Legislature for POW/MIA affairs.

"He worked diligently and was responsible for getting the POW/MIA flag flown in Veteran's Park, and also instrumental in getting the park name changed from Boulder Park to Veteran's Park.

"He worked so hard, and was so dedicated to his missing brothers. He responded to every piece of information and investigation, with the last being Senator John Kerry's visit to Vietnam.

"In our last conversation with him, he said that our government has apparently 'blown off' any further investigation into the POW/MIA matter.

"On January 26, 1993, Bob Stephens took his own life. Lest we forget Bob and our missing brothers, please pick up where he left off. Don't let our government forget. Bob will be greatly missed, but not forgotten."

American Prisoners Of War
Department Of Veteran Affairs, Washington, D.C.

"Some 142,250 Americans were captured and interned during World War I, World War II, the Korean Conflict, the Vietnam Conflict, and the Persian Gulf War. This includes 81 women seized on Guam or in the Philippines in World War II, and two in the Persian Gulf War.

"Of that total, an estimated 66,767 were living as of January 1, 1993, according to Charles A. Stenger of the American Ex-Prisoners of War Association. This includes 90 from World War I, 62,934 from World War II, 3,130 from the Korean Conflict, 590 from the Vietnam Conflict, and 23 from the Persian Gulf War."

	Captured & Interned	Repatriated	Died while POW	Alive January '93
WW1	4,120	3,973	147	90
WWII	130,201	116,129	14,072	62,934
Korea	7,140	4,418	2,701	3,130
Vietnam	766	658	292	590
Gulf	23	23	0	23
TOTAL	142,250	125,201	17,212	66,767

POW/MIA NEWS:
Published by the American Defense Institute:

Long Island Newsday, November 10, 1992 . . . Fearing A New Cover-Up on POW/MIAs . . . .

"Documents unearthed by the Senate Select Committee further established that the U.S. Intelligence Community and the White House knew that a number of servicemen were still alive as recently as 1989.

"For over two decades, both Hanoi and Washington have told uncounted lies to preserve the fiction that everyone who didn't come home was dead."

Thomas Bearpaw:
- POW.
- WWII, U.S. Army with Darby's Rangers.

"I really do not have the answers to these questions. I know what POWs go through because I was one. Out of 1,000 Rangers, the Germans killed all but about 100 and I was one of those.

"I was one of six in my Ranger Company to survive a deadly Nazi counter-attack at Cisterna, Italy; one of three who lived to tell of a disastrous raid on San Peitro, Italy; and an escapee from a POW camp.

"We were captured and marched all over Europe. We survived the 'Black Death March' that took place when the Germans marched American POWs from Poland to Germany. Many died in that march. I have three pictures of U.S. POWs marching by the Roman Wall that was taken by Germans in 1944.

"Maybe my son, George Waite Bearpaw, might know the answers. He was with the 5th Special Forces in Vietnam.

"We had one son in the Korean War and two sons in the Vietnam War."

Dick Cheney:
- Former Secretary of Defense.

"President Bush and his entire Administration were deeply committed to resolving the POW/MIA issue. Returning any Americans who may still be held against their will, obtaining the fullest possible accounting for those still missing and repatriating all recoverable remains of Americans who died serving our Nation during the Vietnam War are objectives of highest national priority for the United States.

"Implementing this shared commitment, the Department of Defense has significantly increased the resources dedicated to this goal. The past year has seen a sweeping expansion in our efforts DoD-wide. From the formation of the office of the Deputy Assistant Secretary of Defense for POW/MIA Affairs, to the activation of the 150-member-strong Joint Task Force-Full Accounting, we have more than doubled the manpower and resources dedicated in resolving this issue.

"This past year also witnessed the establishment of U.S. POW/MIA offices in Hanoi, Vientiane, and Phnom Penh. These in-country offices provide us unprecedented opportunities to press for full implementation of agreements reached with the three Indochinese countries. Our specialists have been allowed to conduct rapid live-sighting investigations and have gained increased access to Vietnam's extensive wartime records. However, much remains to be done.

"Agreements for expanded cooperation are encouraging, but we recognize that results must increase. Government-to-government cooperation is the best means yet found to generate the long overdue answers. At the same time, we also understand that results are the only measure for determining real success.

"The President's resolve is clear. It is with just such unqualified dedication that the men and women of the DoD will continue to strive toward achieving the goal of the fullest possible accounting of those who are still missing. We believe that our missing comrades, their families, and the American people deserve no less."

Roger A. Munson:
• National Commander of the American Legion.
Letters to President Bush
November 6, 1992

Dear Mr. President:
The American Legion is extremely concerned about today's reports that the United States is looking at the possibility of stepping up the pace of the process to recognize Vietnam.

Japan's announcement that it will expand its economic ties with Vietnam and extend large amounts of loans should not be an encouragement to your administration to lift the economic embargo on Vietnam or normalize relations with that country.

The sole criteria for taking such actions should be the degree of Hanoi's cooperation with the U.S. government in resolving the POW/MIA issue.

We find it extremely distressing that Japan, for whom the American taxpayers have provided national defense for four decades, should believe that it is justified in breaking faith with its allies and making a major leap over the wall isolating Vietnam.

In the long run, The American Legion will have no quarrel with lifting the embargo and recognizing the Vietnamese government, but only after we have received total satisfactory cooperation on the POW/MIA issue and have resolved the fate of the missing American servicemen, to the fullest extent possible.

Hanoi's recent partial opening of its archives does not resolve the POW/MIA issue. It is a welcome step, although it was over 20 years late in coming. Too often in the past, Hanoi's broad promises of POW/MIA cooperation have turned out in the end to have been empty gestures aimed at the gullible.

In the strongest possible terms, the more than 3.1 million members of the American Legion call upon you to 'hold the line' against Hanoi and not take any favorable action on expanding economic relations, lifting the economic embargo or normalizing relations until our POW/MIAs have been accounted for and the anguish of POW/MIA families has been ended.

Roger A. Munson

November 19, 1992

Dear Mr. President:

On behalf of the nation's largest veterans' organization, the American Legion, I strongly urge you not to take any further steps toward the diplomatic recognition of Vietnam or the lifting of the trade embargo at this point in time.

We are alarmed at the fact you saw fit to write a letter to President Le Duc Anh of Vietnam wherein, according to press reports, you promised 'reciprocal actions' toward Hanoi for their perceived cooperative efforts on the POW/MIA issue.

It appears your administration is on the verge of being stampeded into taking unwise and unjustified favorable action toward Vietnam based on the flimsiest possible evidence of increased cooperation.

Not all of the material made available by the Vietnamese Communists in recent days is new. Some of the material was viewed by a member of our staff during a briefing at the Army Museum in Hanoi more than a year ago.

Its highly promoted release at this time seems to be a cleverly calculated move by Hanoi to capitalize on the impending change in administrations. However, we have serious reservations as to just how helpful these photographs and war relics will be in actually resolving any significant number of POW/MIA cases.

We are frustrated at having been told for 12 years that the POW/MIA issue is of the highest national priority, when in reality, during the last three administrations only minimal progress has been achieved despite much rhetoric.

Based on the current scenario the American Legion can only conclude that the termination of the Senate Select Committee on POW/MIA Affairs will occur, issuance of an incomplete report by that body appears inevitable, and either total or partial lifting of the embargo and a move toward normalization of relations will occur.

We call on you once again to "hold the line" on favorable actions toward Vietnam. To do otherwise, before achieving real progress in resolving the POW/MIA issue, is to forfeit the only leverage the United States has in fulfilling its moral obligations to the missing American servicemen and their families.

Roger A. Munson

December 14, 1992

Dear Mr. President:

Once again, the more than 3.1 million members of the American Legion want to make sure you understand our complete opposition to premature moves toward lifting the economic embargo and normalization of relations with Vietnam. We are utterly disappointed and totally outraged at your announcement permitting signing of contracts in Vietnam and easing licensing restrictions.

Vietnam's "cooperation" on the POW/MIA issue has been mostly rhetorical and has not provided concrete results. U.S. government officials have recently advised us that, thus far, Hanoi has provided only about one percent of the information that is available.

To reiterate what was stated, in part, in my last letter to you dated November 19, 1992, The American Legion has serious reservations as to how helpful the recently released photographs and war relics will be in actually resolving any significant number of POW/MIA cases. Your practice of giving Hanoi great rewards for minimal actions is a certain way to ensure that the fullest possible POW/MIA accounting will never be achieved.

From its very misguided inception, the "road map" has been a recipe for letting the Communist leaders of Vietnam evade their responsibilities under the Paris Peace Accords of 1973 to return all American POWs.

As your administration enters its final days, we strongly urge you, as we did in our letter to you of November 19, to "hold the line" on taking favorable actions toward Hanoi.

After Vietnam provides the fullest possible accounting for our POW/MIAs, then, and only then, will it be the proper time to reward the Vietnamese with the economic benefits they so desperately need. Any other course of action will be to desert the POW/MIAs and their families in their time of greatest need.

So, an important question still hovers over the government and the families of the missing like a dark cloud. What remains of the POW/MIA issue?

Roger A. Munson

National Commander Robert A. Munson told *The American Legion* magazine that, "Senator John McCain of Arizona, a Vietnam veteran and former POW, got his flight helmet back from the Socialist Republic of Vietnam, thanks to the Senate Select Committee on POW/MIA Affairs."

McCain's helmet, along with thousands of photographs and a collection of U.S. Vietnam-era combat gear, appear to be all a $1.9 million, 14-month investigation could pry from the Communists in Vietnam.

In the words of committee Vice Chairman Senator Robert C. Smith of New Hampshire, a Vietnam veteran, "It's nice to have Sen. McCain's helmet, but John McCain is home."

The committee's investigation of the POW/MIA issue both succeeded and failed.

It succeeded in establishing that the truth about our POW/MIAs has never been told, either by the U.S. government or by the Vietnamese.

It failed in that it discovered enough to prove we were living a lie, but it didn't uncover the truth.

We applaud the committee for making unprecedented progress in declassifying POW/MIA documents and intelligence. More information is available today than ever before. But much more needs to be made public.

We were encouraged by the committee's ability to move the issue further into public view through a series of revealing hearings.

And we're pleased that the committee took our recommendation and had the U.S. Army's Central Identification Laboratory in Hawaii (CIL-HI) investigated. In the past, CIL-HI has done a poor job in identifying remains. And despite new leadership, there is a long road ahead toward credibility.

If we compare what the committee accomplished with what it set out to do—mainly to determine if live POWs were still captive in Southeast Asia, Russia, Korea or China—the investigation, overall, is disappointing.

Were there American POWs left behind in Southeast Asia after the Vietnam War? If so, why were they left behind and who left them there? Could any of these men still be alive?

For nearly 20 years, the U.S. government has answered these questions with one word: "No."

The committee only answered one of these questions: Americans were left behind. But who left them and whether or not they are alive today remains an open question.

Ambiguous signals gradually began to emerge from the committee indicating that the investigation had run its course. Some senators, it seemed, were content with the committee's accomplishments and were prepared to close the book on the POW/MIA investigation.

After returning from a trip to Vietnam, Senator John F. Kerry of Massachusetts, the committee chairman, began calling for the U.S. economic embargo to be lifted before the probe was completed. He suggested that Vietnam be "rewarded" for its cooperation.

The committee is tasked with answering questions on the fate of our missing, not with making foreign policy. Why was Kerry overstepping his authority?

This was particularly disturbing in light of Garnett E. Bell's 1991 testimony. Bell, former chief of the U.S. Office of POW/MIA Affairs in Hanoi, testified that the U.S. government had "information of Americans being held" after Operation Homecoming—after all U.S. POWs were said to be returned. Bell added that there was "hard evidence" that at least 10 Americans were left behind.

Former Defense Secretaries James R. Schlesinger and Melvin R. Laird supported Bell's testimony that Americans were left behind. Not only did the committee fail to determine if there are live U.S. POWs still in captivity, but it also failed to find out who left them there.

If these Senate hearings are taken as one step in the development of a new POW/MIA policy, then they should be considered a small success. They have both elevated the issue and ended some of the secrecy. If, however, the committee's work is used to close the book on our POW/MIAs, then we have learned very little.

Miles Z. Epstein:
• Editor, *The American Legion* magazine.

"How can America protect its captured and missing military personnel in future wars? How can America be sure no one is left behind? According to experts, these nine steps can bring our people home:

1. **"Let the world know that our resolve to bring all Americans home includes diplomatic sanctions, economic embargoes and military retaliation.**

"'Anytime an American is seized or killed, we should take physical retribution for that act,' says retired Adm. Thomas H. Moorer, former chairman of the Joint Chiefs of Staff (1970-1974). 'We've set a precedent that the United States will do nothing.

"'By retaliating, we are not risking lives just to save one man,' Moorer explains, 'but ensuring that no more Americans are ever taken. I think it's worth going to war over.'

2. **"Establish rules of engagement for war and peacekeeping that protect prisoners and missing.**

"It has been said that no plan survives contact with the enemy. But just as formal declarations of war seem to be a thing of the past, so do traditional military operations.

"Since Congress has declared peacekeeping and humanitarian assistance to be 'valid military missions,' the U.S. Armed Forces are now being deployed without a plan or an enemy. No plan. No enemy. No protection for prisoners or missing.

"How can America protect the troops it sends into undeclared wars, or on peacekeeping or humanitarian missions? Rules of engagement are needed.

Retired Army Col. Harry Summers, Jr. opposes peacekeeping and humanitarian missions for the military in principle.

"'The armed forces shouldn't be used as a signaling device,' Summers says. He states that the United States should let the military do what it was designed for, 'fight wars.'

"The United States needs to be sure POW status is given to troops who are taken during peacekeeping and humanitarian operations. Or it should follow Summers' advice, and keep U.S. forces out of combat engagements if they cannot be protected.

3. "Centralize intelligence to keep track of those in combat, captured or missing.

"'The American intelligence community has to be reorganized,' former Delta Force Commander Paschall says. 'It needs to be made more responsive to American needs.'

"From Vietnam to Desert Storm, the agencies that collected intelligence have often not known what to do with it. And, it appears, this has jeopardized the lives of POWs and MIAs.

"'People died in Vietnam because POW/MIA intelligence was so highly-classified, and it didn't get to the right people,' says Jerry Mooney.

4. "Treat the hunt for POW/MIAs as an unresolved crime.

"Getting good intelligence isn't worth anything if it isn't used properly. And when it comes to POW/MIA information, this is a big problem.

"Basic police work has not been done on most POW/MIA cases. Experts, like Eugene Tighe, say that this must change.

"'In bloody and prolonged battle, we tend to start talking about statistics,' Tighe says. 'That's wrong. We've got to stop talking about numbers and start talking about names. Only then can we start bringing missing Americans home.'

5. "Offer asylum to foreign citizens who help recover POWs.

"House bill H.R. 1900, had it passed, would have 'granted asylum in the United States to nationals of Laos, Vietnam, Cambodia and Burma who assisted in the return of live American POW/MIAs from Indochina.'

"The failure of the bill was tragic in view of the high-ranking Vietnamese official, Nguyen Can, who sought to defect with information on live prisoners, but instead was recalled to Vietnam before he could do so.

"What happened to Mr. Can?

"After returning to Vietnam, Can disappeared and many fear he's been locked away by his government or killed. 'We should demand to see Mr. Can,' Senator Smith told *The American Legion* magazine.

"Many experts believe that if America doesn't guarantee protection to foreign citizens who help recover live U.S. POWs, no one will come forward with information.

"For Vietnam and for future wars, we need to encourage—even reward—foreign citizens who help bring home Americans.

6. "End the secrecy on the POW/MIA issue.

"Testifying before the Senate, acting assistant Secretary of Defense for International Security Affairs Carl W. Ford pledged an end to secrecy.

"'Our ability to continue to collect information for the families and for other intelligence projects requires us to try to keep our sources and methods protected,' Ford explained. 'We've used that many more times than I would like to admit as an excuse, rather than as a real answer. I'm simply telling you that it's over. We're going to find a way to do this.'

7. "Set up a group that really helps POW/MIA families.

"'The kind of assets that we have now applied against the problem (POW/MIAs) would have been best applied then (20 years ago). I can't recover from that, and I can't apologize enough to the families personally,' Dennis Nagy, acting DIA director, told the Senate committee.

8. "Provide theater commanders with well-trained and well-equipped combat search and rescue forces.

"The best way to prevent a downed pilot or stranded infantryman from becoming a POW is to rescue him before he's captured. Combat search and rescue (CSAR) should be a national priority. Theater commanders must call the shots on CSAR. In Desert Storm, this mistake was not repeated. CSAR was directed by the Joint Commander.

9. "Appoint a permanent presidential commission or congressionally-approved government board on POW/MIAs to recommend, plan and monitor.

"'America needs to set up a policy that won't allow POWs to be abandoned in future wars,' says National Commander Munson. 'And the first step is to move the process out of the Pentagon and the intelligence community.'

"Retired Army General Vessey agrees. 'I have recommended that the President set up a review body to look at what is being done on the POW issue, and find out how to do it better,' says Vessey.

"'It's not enough to move heaven and earth, you have to move hell,' says retired Adm. Thomas H. Moorer, former chairman of the Joint Chiefs of Staff. And to Moorer, that means going to war, if necessary, to bring our men home."

Part 3

My spirit shakes with terror;
How long, O Lord, how long?

Psalms 6:3

Statistics

Confusion reigns when it comes to numbers and the Vietnam War. Listed below are some figures that may help sort fact from fiction in many media reports.

- 9,087,000 military personnel served on active duty during the Vietnam era (Aug. 5, 1964–May 7, 1975).

- 8,744,000 personnel were on active duty during the war (Aug. 5, 1964–March 28, 1973).

- 3,403,100 (including 514,300 offshore) personnel served in the Southeast Asia Theater (Vietnam, Laos, Cambodia, flight crews based in Thailand, and sailors in adjacent South China Sea waters).

- 2,594,000 personnel served within the borders of South Vietnam (Jan. 1, 1965–March 28, 1973).

- Another 50,000 men served in Vietnam between 1960 and 1964.

- Of the 2.6 million, between 1 million and 1.6 million (40–60 percent) either fought in combat, provided close combat support or were at least fairly regularly exposed to enemy attack.

- 7,484 women (6,250 or 83.5 percent were nurses) served in Vietnam.

- Peak troop strength in Vietnam: 543,482 (April 30, 1969).

- There were 58,156 casualties (including men formerly classified as MIA and Mayaguez Casualties). Twenty-seven other men have died of wounds, bringing the total to 58,183.

- 8 nurses died—1 was killed in action. There were 17,539 married men KIA and 61 percent of the men killed were 21 years old or younger. The average age of the Vietnam veteran was 19 (26 for WWII).

- 2,338 were missing in action and there were 766 prisoners of war (114 died in captivity). There were 303,704 wounded in action.

- 82 percent of the veterans who saw heavy combat strongly believe the war was lost because of lack of political will.

- Nearly 75 percent of the general public agrees that it was a failure of political will, not of arms.

- 91 percent of actual Vietnam War veterans and 90 percent of those who saw heavy combat are proud to have served their country.

- 66 percent of Vietnam veterans say they would serve again if called upon.

- 87 percent of the public now holds Vietnam veterans in high esteem.

Of the major U.S. combat unit casualties in Vietnam, the units listed below account for 98 percent of the Americans killed or wounded by hostile action in Vietnam.

Unit	KIA	Wounded
III Marine Amphibious Force	13,082	26,592
1st Marine Division		
1st Marine Aircraft Wing		
3rd Marine Division		
7th Fleet Amphibious Force		
1st Cavalry Division	5,444	26,592
25th Infantry Division	4,547	31,161
101st Airborne Division	4,011	18,259
1st Infantry Division	3,146	18,019
9th Infantry Division	2,624	18,831
4th Infantry Division	2,531	15,229
173rd Airborne Division	1,748	8,747
7th Air Force/SAC (Guam)	1,739	3,457
1st Aviation Brigade	1,701	5,163
7th Fleet/Naval Forces	1,826	10,406
196th Light Inf. Brigade	1,004	5,591
America (23rd) Division	808	8,237
11th Light Infantry Brigade		
198th Light Infantry Brigade		
199th Light Infantry Brigade	754	4,679
11th Armored Cavalry Regime	728	5,671
5th Special Forces Group	645	2,704
5th Mech. Infantry Division	403	3,648
1st Brigade		
82nd Airborne Division	184	1,009
3rd Brigade		
Coast Guard Squadrons 1 and 3	5	59

Part 4

Rescue me from my enemies, O God:
Protect me from those who rise up against me!

Psalms 5:9

Dear Mr. Robertson;

President Clinton and I share your concern about Americans who are missing and unaccounted for in Southeast Asia. As a Vietnam veteran, I have very strong personal feelings about this issue. While in the Senate, I supported the creation of the Senate Select Committee on POW/MIA affairs to fully investigate this matter.

The government of Vietnam has committed to unilaterally conducting a country-wide search of all its archives for documents, photographs and other materials related to American POW/MIA cases and will make all such material available to us at its military museums. The government of Vietman also has agreed to form a joint information research team to examine all of these materials. We believe that this activity will help us to determine the fate of many American POW/MIAs.

Obtaining the fullest possible accounting for our missing servicemen remains the most important objective of our policy toward Vietnam. Please be assured that President Clinton and I place the highest national priority on returning anyone who may may still be held captive, accounting for those still missing, and repatriating recoverable remains of those who died serving our nation.

Sincerely,
Al Gore
Vice President

List of Unaccounted For POW/MIAs

Prepared by the Office of Senator Bob Smith Vice Chairman, Senate Select Committee on POW/MIA Affairs, this listing contains the names of 324 still unaccounted for U.S. personnel from the Vietnam Conflict.

Approximately 300 of these personnel were last known alive in captivity in Vietnam and Laos, last known alive, out of their aircraft before it crashed, or their names were passed to POWs who later returned. A handful of the cases involves incidents when the aircraft was later found on the ground with no sign of the crew.

This listing is based on all-source U.S. intelligence and casualty reports, information provided by POWs who were returned, lists of POWs and/or last-known alive personnel prepared by the Defense Intelligence Agency, and other information made available to the Vice Chairman, Select Committee on POW/MIA Affairs.

The difference between 300 and 324 personnel accounts for known incidents when one or more unidentified crew members were captured from a crew of more than one, or the aircraft was found with no trace of the crew.

Based on the high number of unaccounted for MIAs at the end of the war (currently 1,170 persons for whom the USG does not know their fate), it is probable that a significant percentage of those not on this list actually survived their incident and could have been captured.

Apparently, only the Vietnamese and Laotians would know their fate, as the U.S. government does not. Given this reality, the list of 324 names which follows is, at best, conservative.

Moreover, it should be noted that this number is consistent with the overall numbers represented in the volume of detailed eyewitness and hearsay accounts of reported U.S. POWs in captivity following the war in Vietnam and Laos which have been the focus of investigation by the committee staff.

This is a working document expected to be revised and updated as selected MIA files, eyewitness and hearsay post-war POW reports, special

intelligence, returnee debriefs, and other information continues to be analyzed by the vice chairman.

Acosta-Rosario, Humberto
USA—Last known alive, DoD April 1991 list.

Adam, John G.
USAF—Laos, name mentioned by Soviet correspondent. (NSA intercept
correlation.)

Adams, Lee Aaron
USAF—Hearsay secondhand knowledge of Adams survival provided by POW
returnee Michael L. Brazelton.

Algard, Harold L.
USA—Possibly captured alive according to NSA intercept correlation.
(Intercept—three out of five from JU21A incident alive and captured.)

Allard, Richard M.
USA—POW identified by family members in Viet Cong film clips. Mother
claims to Associated Press (3-9-73) to have been allowed to see Allard in NVN
prison camp in Cambodia. (See AP story 3-9-73.)

Alinson, David J.
USAF—Good chute observed.

Anderson, Gregory Lee
USAF—Beeper heard for short period. DIA analytical comment, 1979.

Anderson, Robert D.
USAF—Believed to have ejected from aircraft according to POW Returnee
Latella debrief L079.

Andrews, William R.
USAF—Voice contact made on ground, wounded. DIA analytical comment,
979. POW according to secondhand hearsay information obtained through
prison communication. (See POW Returnee Brady and Talley debriefs,
B096 and T001.)

Ard, Randolph J.
USA—Laos, out of aircraft before crash. (JTF-FA Survival Code 1.)

Armstrong, John W.
USAF—Laos, known captured. Interviewed by Soviet correspondent.
(NSA intercept correlation.)

Ashlock, Carlos
USMC—Last known alive, DoD April 1991 list.

Avery, Robert D.
USMC—POW according to passed down list. POW early returnee Norris
Charles memorized a list of reported prisoners which included Avery's full name.

Ayers, Richard L.
USAF—Laos, possible correlation as POW in Cu Loc and Zoo prisons according
to hearsay information provided by POW returnee Leo Hyat H097. Shoot-down of
aircraft confirmed by Hanoi radio with no mention of fate of crew.

Babula, Robert L.
USMC—Last known alive, DoD April 1991 list.

Backus, Kenneth F.
USAF—Believed to have successfully exited of his aircraft and was alive on the ground. Last known alive, DoD April 1991 list.

Baker, Arthur D.
USAF—Laos, believed to have successfully exited of his aircraft and was alive on the ground. Last known alive, DoD April 1991 list.

Balcom, Ralph C.
USAF—Laos, exited aircraft before crash. (JTF-FA Survival Code 1.)

Bancroft, William W.
USAF—Possibly captured according to NSA intercept correlation. (One known captured from crew of two.)

Bannon, Paul W.
USAF—Laos, possible correlation to live-sighting information and intelligence pertaining to 1981 Nhom Marrot activities. (25 June 1981 Defense Department closed-door testimony.)

Barden, Howard L.
USAF—Laos, Survival possible, DIA 1979 report.

Begley, Burriss N.
USAF—Name scratched on floor at Ha Lo prison. (See Stutz debrief 123.) Last-known direct voice contact with Begley was during incident when Begley stated he was ejecting from his aircraft.

Bennett, William G.
USAF—POW according to secondhand info. Reported as prisoner on Hanoi radio broadcast. (See Overly debrief.)

Bodenschatz, John E.
USMC—Last known alive, DoD April 1991 list.

Bogiages, Christos C.
USAF—Laos, exited aircraft before crash. (JTF-FA Survival Code 1.)

Borah, Daniel V.
USN—Hostile capture, (DoD June, 1973 list) believed to have successfully exited his aircraft and was alive on the ground. Last known alive, DoD April 1991 list. Known captured according to NSA intercept correlation.

Borton, Robert C.
USMC—Last known alive, DoD April 1991 list.

Bouchard, Michael
USN—Laos, possible POW in good health according to notes obtained in prison by POW returnee Roger Miller. The name "Boucher" was passed.

Bram, Richard, C.
USMC—Last known alive, DoD April 1991 list. Reported as POW by SVN Pol. (DIA 1979 report).

Brandenberg, Dale
USAF–Laos, EC47Q, Baron 52, believed to have been captured according to analysts in 1973 based on NSA intelligence reports.

Brashear, William J.
USAF–Laos, exited aircraft before crash. (JTF-FA Survival Code 1.) Believed to have successfully gotten out of his aircraft and was alive on the ground. Last known alive, DoD April 1991 list.

Brennan, Herbert O.
USAF–Believed to have successfully exited his aircraft and was alive on the ground. Last known alive, DoD April 1991 list.

Breuer, Donald C.
USMC–Laos, good parachute reported by enemy; enemy reports they are attempting capture according to NSA intercept correlation.

Brown, George R.
USA–Laos, known to be alive on the ground during helicopter exfiltration. When the rope ladder broke and hostile forces approached, the helicopter departed leaving Brown and Hurston, alive and unwounded. Search team inserted four days later. No sign of Brown or Huston. (JCRC report.)

Brown, Harry W.
USA–Last known alive, DoD April 1991 list.

Brown, Robert M.
USAF–Laos/NVN, captured alive according to same-day intelligence report indication capture of pilots of a low-flying aircraft in same location and giving orders to "conceal the accomplishment." (No other shootdowns correlate to this report.) Intelligence report one week later requested special Vietnamese team to transport the hulk of a F-111. NSA analyst recalls Brown on list of POWs moved to Sam Neua for movement to USSR. Brown's military ID card has surfaced in good condition at military museum in Vinh. NVN defector states intact portion of F-111 sent to China same month as Brown shootdown, NVN photographers not allowed to keep photos of the F-111.

Brownlee, Charles R.
USAF–Laos, exited aircraft before crash. (JTF-FA Survival Code 1.)

Brownlee, Robert W.
USA–Evaded on ground with RVN Lt. (POW Returnee William Reeder debrief.)

Brucher, John M.
USAF–Voice contact made, injured in parachute in tree. DIA report, 1979. Last known alive, DoD April 1991 list.

Buckley, Louis
USA–Last known alive, DoD April 1991 list.

Buell, Kenneth R.
USN–Possibly captured according to NSA intercept correlation. (One pilot captured from incident.)

Bunker, Park G.
USAF–Laos, out of aircraft before crash. (JTF-FA Survival Code 1.)

Burnett, Sheldon J.
USA—Laos, out of aircraft before crash. (JTF-FA Survival Code 1.)

Bynum, Neil S.
USAF—Laos, one pilot parachuted and probably captured according to NSA intercept correlation. (F4D-two seater.)

Carlock, Ralph L.
USAF—Laos, POW, captured by Pathet Lao forces according to FBIS intercept PL radio communication.
Believed to have successfully exited his aircraft and was alive on the ground. Last known alive, DoD April 1991 list.

Carr, Donald Gene
USA—Laos, reported as POW. (DoD DOI report, July 1971.)

Carroll, John L.
USAF—Laos, out of aircraft before crash. (JTF-FA Survival Code 1.)

Carter, Dennis R.
USMC—Last known alive, DoD April 1991 list.

Champion, James A.
USA—Survived helicopter crash and was observed walking away from site in good physical condition armed with an M-16 rifle. M154 debrief.

Chestnut, Joseph, L.
USAF—Laos, out of aircraft before crash. (JTF-FA Survival Code 1.)
Captured according to NVN records. (Source: Bob Destatte, Bill Bell, JTF-FA.)
Sighted alive in captivity after the war. (Source: Bill Bell, JTF-FA.)

Cichon, Walter A.
USA—Possibly captured according to DIA analytical comment, 1979.
Last known alive, DoD April 1991 list. Listed as POW by DIA, 1973. NSA correlation as captured. Wartime ralliers reported Cichon as captured (DIA 1992 analytical comment). U.S. field investigation has identified Vietnamese witness who states Cichon was captured and transferred to higher authorities.

Clark, Richard C.
USN—Good chute observed. (DIA analytical comment, 1979.) Hostile capture (DoD June 1973 list). Listed as POW by DIA, 1973. Name on memorized list of POWs according to information from POW returnee C.P. Zuhoski.

Clark, Fred L.
USAF—Laos, one parachute observed from mid-air collision, possible correlation. (DIA report, 1979.)

Clarke, George W.
USAF—Laos/VN, hostile capture. (DoD June 1973 list.) Listed as POW by DIA, 1973. Last known alive, Laos DoD April 1991 list.

Coady, Robert F.
USAF—Laos, hearsay POW. Rumble debrief. (DIA Oct. 3, 1969, State Sept. 25, 1969.)

Cohron, James D.
USA–Laos, last known alive, DoD April 1991 list.

Collamore, Allan P.
USN–Firsthand contact by tap code in prison system made by POW
returnee James Mulligan.

Condit, Douglas C.
USAF–Believed to have successfully exited his aircraft and was alive on the
ground. Last known alive, DoD April 1991 list.

Cook, Dwight W.
USAF–Identified as POW by Thai returnees, 1973. Possibly captured
according to NSA intercept correlation.

Cook, Kely F.
USAF–Believed to have successfully exited his aircraft and was alive on the
ground. Last known alive, DoD April 1991 list.

Cornwell, Leroy J.
USAF–Laos, name reported by POW returnee Arthur Cormier (JSSA).

Cramer, Donald R.
USA–Name passed on a note in Cu Loc/Zoo prison according to POW
Returnee Charles. Name in the POW memory bank according to POW
Returnees Jeffrey and Charles.

Creed, Barton S.
USN–Laos, voice contact on ground, DIA 1973. "May have been
captured," DIA report 1973. JTF-FA Survival Code 1 (March 13, 1992). Listed as
POW by DIA, 1973. Last known alive, DoD April 1991 list. NSA intercept
correlation.

Cressman, Peter R.
USAF–Laos, EC47Q, Baron 52, believed to have been captured according to
analysts in 1973 based on NSA intelligence reports.

Crew, James A.
USAF–Believed to have successfully exited his aircraft and was alive on the
ground. Last known alive, DoD April 1991 list.

Cristman, Frederick L.
USA–Laos, exited aircraft before crash. (JTF-FA Survival Code 1.)

Crockett, William J.
USAF–Possibly captured according to NSA intercept correlation. (One pilot
captured from two-seater aircraft.)

Cushman, Clifton E.
USAF–POW according to hearsay information obtained by POW returnees
Hyatt (HO97 debrief). Name mentioned in French news report following
incident.

Cuthbert, Bradley G.
USAF–Seen alive in good chute (according to Ruhling debrief RO53).
Believed to have successfully exited his aircraft and was alive,
DoD April 1991 list.

Dahill, Douglas E.

USA—Last known alive, DoD April 1991 list.

Dale, Charles A.

USA—Last known alive, DoD April 1991 list.

Danielson, Benjamin F.

USAF—Laos, exited aircraft before crash. (JTF-FA Survival Code 1.)

Davies, Joseph E.

USAF—Believed to be alive according to prison communication information obtained by POW returnee Mulligan. (M131 debrief.)

Davidson, David A.

USA— Laos, captured alive by enemy forces according to NSA/DIA intercept correlation.

Davis, Edgar F.

USAF—Laos, exited aircraft before crash. (JTF-FA Survival Code 1.)

Debruin, Eugene H.

Laos—pilot of C-46. Shown alive in photo.

DeLong, Joe L.

USA—listed as POW by DIA (Cat.3) (January 31, 1992 deposition).

Demmon, David S.

USA—Hostile capture (DoD June 1973 list)—listed as POW by DIA. 1973.—Last known alive, DoD April 1991 list.

Dexter, Bennie L.

USAF—POW capture witnessed. DIA 1979 report—hostile capture, (DoD June 1973 list)—last known alive, DoD April 1991 list. Hearsay information obtained by POW returnee Donald Rander (R047).

Dickson, Edward A.

USN—Ejected from aircraft DIA analytical comment, 1979.

Dinan, David T.

USAF—Laos, exited aircraft before crash. (JTF-FA Survival Code 1)

Dingwell, John F.

USMC—Possible POW according to SVN Pol., search negative. DIA Report, 1979.—Last known alive, DoD April 1991 list.

Dodge, Edward R.

USA—Last known alive, DoD April 1991 list.

Donahue, Morgan

USAF—One parachute observed from mid-air collision, Donahue subject of subsequent live-sighting reports (CIA-DIA).

Dooley, James E.

USN—Identified as POW Thai returnee, 1973. POW Returnee Daugherty heard that his name had been seen on wall. (Daugherty debrief.)

Duckett, Thomas A.

USAF—Laos, exited aircraft before crash. (JTF-FA Survival Code 1.)

Dunlop, Thomas E.
USN—Believed to have successfully exited his aircraft and was alive on the ground. Last known alive, DoD April 1991 list.

Dunn, Michael E.
USN—Believed to have successfully exited his aircraft and was alive on the ground. Last known alive, DoD April 1991 list.

Edwards, Harry S.
USN—Possibly a POW according to hearsay information in the prison system. (Flom, Mahoney debriefs.)

Egan, James T.
USMC—Last known alive, DoD April 1991 list.

Eidsmoe, Norman E.
USN—POW according to secondhand information, possibly Son Tay (Naughton debrief). Believed to have successfully exited his aircraft and was alive on the ground. Last known alive, DoD April 1991 list.

Elliott, Robert M.
USAF Captured, POW according to several "reliable" intelligence reports. (NSA/DIA analytical comment.)

Ellis, William
USA—Last known alive, DoD April 1991 list.

Ellison, John C.
USN—Positively identified as a POW in picture shown to POW returnee Robert Flynn by Chinese cadre while in captivity. Ellison appeared in good condition in picture, which showed a group of 10-12 guarded American POWs being marched through a crowd of people. Ellison was in the front row. Ellison's name carved in tree at Dogpatch prison Chinese border according to two unidentified returnees that contacted Ellison's family.

Entrican, Danny D.
USA—Last known alive, DoD April 1991 list. Radio interception indicated Entrican had been captured and was to be moved north to Hanoi according to POW returnee. (See returnee debrief Jon Cavaiani C139.)

Estocin, Michael J.
USN—Possible POW according to secondhand information from Rivers, Mayhew, and Smith debriefs. Hostile capture (DoD June 1973 list). Listed as POW by DIA, 1973. Last known alive, DoD April 1991 list.

Fallon, Patrick M.
USAF—Laos, exited aircraft before crash. (JTF-FA Survival Code 1.)

Finley, Diclie W.
USA—Last known alive, DoD April 1991 list.

Fischer, Richard W.
USMC—Last known alive, DoD April 1991 list.

Fitzgerald, Joseph E.
USA—Last known alive, DoD April 1991 list.

Fitzgerald, Paul L.
USA—Last known alive, DoD April 1991 list.

Fors, Gary H.
USMC—Laos, exited aircraft before crash. (JTF-FA Survival Code 1.)

Foulks, Ralph E.
USN—Possible POW according to returnee Ballard debrief and DIA possible correlation in 1973.

Fowler, Donald R.
USA—Last known alive, DoD April 1991 list.

Francisco, San D.
USAF—Voice contact on ground, DIA report. 1979. POW according to NSA report, November 27, 1968. Listed as POW by DIA, 1973. Last known alive, DoD April 1991 list.

Fryer, Bruce C.
USN—Laos, exited aircraft before crash. (JTF-FA Survival Code 1.)

Gage, Robert H.
USMC—Last known alive, DoD April 1991 list.

Galbraith, Russell D.
USAF—Laos, exited aircraft before crash. (JTF-FA Survival Code 1.)

Gallent, Henry J.
USA—Last known alive, DoD April 1991 list.

Garcia, Ricardo M.
USA—Laos, exited aircraft before crash. (JTF-FA Survival Code 1.)

Gassman, Fred A.
USA—Laos, captured alive by enemy forces according to NSA/DIA intercept correlation.

Gates, James W.
USA—Laos, radio contact on ground. (DIA report) Out of aircraft before crash. (JTF-FA Survival Code 1.) Believed to have successfully exited his aircraft and was alive on the ground. Last known alive, DoD April 1991 list.

Gerstel, Donald A.
USN—Known captured according to NSA intercept correlation.

Glasson, William A.
USN—Down and captured in China according to Peking Bulletin and Peking Radio. Information obtained by POW returnee Phillip Smith.

Gould, Frank A.
USAF—Laos, alive and waiting rescue according to Peter J. Giroux returnee debrief G104. Exited aircraft before crash. (JTF-FA Survival Code 1.) Search and Rescue Team (SAR) reported seeing mirror flashes from area where rest of crew was picked up, but nightfall prevented further rescue attempts (JCRC).

Parachuted into hill, awaiting rescue, voice contact and beeper heard. Ground search on following day found helmet and parachute, but no sign of Gould. Gould is subject of live-sighting reports from Laos in the 1990s. (DIA Stoney Beach reports.)

Grace, James W.

USAF–Laos, exited aircraft before crash. (JTF-FA Survival Code 1.) Attempted rescue unsuccessful. Family member post-capture identification in Communist propaganda film (PL guard).

Graf, John G.

USN–Believed to be alive as POW in Viet Cong-controlled area in 1973 according to POW returnee Robert White. Hostile capture (DoD June 1973 list). Listed as POW by DIA, 1973.

Green, Frank C.

USN–Known captured according to NSA intercept correlation.

Greenleaf, Joseph G.

USN–Believed to have successfully exited his aircraft and was alive on the ground. Last known alive, DoD April 1991 list. One parachute seen according to "generally reliable sources" (DIA analytical comment).

Greenwood, Robert R.

USAF–Laos, POW at "Zoo" prison in Vietnam according to secondhand information. (See Brunhaver B102 debrief.) Exited aircraft before crash. (JTF-FA Survival Code 1.)

Greiling, David S.

USN–POW according to secondhand information. Name heard in system. (Anderson debrief.) Hostile capture (DoD June 1973). Listed as POW by DIA, 1973.

Groth, Wade L.

USA–Last known alive, DoD April 1991 list.

Gunn, Alan W.

USA–Last known alive, DoD April 1991 list.

Hamilton, John S.

USAF–Believed to have successfully exited his aircraft and was alive on the ground. Last known alive, DoD April 1991 list.

Hamilton, Roger D.

USMC–Last known alive, DoD April 1991 list.

Hamm, James E.

USAF–Believed to have successfully exited his aircraft and was alive on the ground. Last known alive, DoD April 1991 list.

Hargrove, Olin

USA–Last known alive, DoD April 1991 list.

Harris, Jeffrey L.

USAF–Possibly captured according to NSA intercept correlation.

Harris, Reuben B.
USN—Crew down and captured in China according to Peking Bulletin and Peking Radio. Information obtained by POW returnee Phillip Smith.

Harrison, Donald L.
USA—POW according to POW Returnee Wesley Rumble—based on secondhand list.

Hasenback, Paul A.
USA—Last known alive, DoD April 1991 list.

Hastings, Steven M.
USA—Last known alive, DoD April 1991 list.

Held, John W.
USAF—Believed to have successfully exited his aircraft and was alive on the ground. Last known alive, DoD April 1991 list.

Helwig, Roger D.
USAF—Laos, exited aircraft before crash. (JTF-FA Survival Code 1.)

Hentz, Richard J.
USA—Possibly captured alive according to NSA intercept correlation. (Intercept—three out of five from JU21A incident alive and captured.)

Herold, Richard W.
USAF—Laos, exited aircraft before crash. (JTF-FA Survival Code 1.)

Hesford, Peter D.
USAF—Laos, believed to have successfully exited his aircraft and was alive on the ground. Last known alive, DoD April 1991 list.

Hess, Frederick W.
USAF—Laos, exited aircraft before crash. (JTF-FA Survival Code 1.)

Hestle, Roosevelt
USAF—Seen alive at Heartbreak prison, possibly tortured and carried on stretcher. (Bolstad debrief, BO91.) Believed to have successfully exited his aircraft and was alive on the ground. Last known alive, DoD April 1991 list.

Hicks, Terrin D.
USAF—Believed to have been captured alive and taken to Dong Hoi for medical treatment of a broken leg, according to information from POW returnee debriefs. (Uyeyama and Shanahan, U004 and S021.)

Hodgson, Cecil J.
USA—Last known alive, DoD April 1991 list.

Holland, Melvin A.
USAF—Laos, possibly captured, based on report the following day by Thai survivor of Lima Site 85 incident, and comments by former PL General Singkapo in 1991, whose subsequent recanting remains suspect. (Both sources stated three Americans were captured by NVN troops during the incident.)

Holley, Tilden S.
USAF—POW according to hearsay information obtained by returning POWs Ellis, Fisher and Heiliger—(See debriefs EO28, FO45, and HO85.) Ellis reported full name. Possibly held in Cu Loc and the Zoo prisons.

Holmes, David H.
USAF–Laos, exited aircraft before crash. (JTF-FA Survival Code 2.) Search and Rescue unable to locate pilot. (DIA 1979 report.)

Holmes, Frederick L.
USN–POW believed to have been held at Cu Loc and Zoo prisons. (Kiern debrief, K046.) Known to have ejected from aircraft. (Source: DIA analytical comment.)

Hrdlicka, David L.
USAF–POW in Laos, voice recording and (P.L.)Pathet Lao/*Pravda* photograph including his name. Letter signed by Hrdlicka while in captivity appeared in NVN/PL magazine.

Hubert, Eric J.
USAF–Cambodia, possibly captured according to NSA intercept correlation. (F4D two-seater, one known captured.)

Hunt, Robert W.
USA–Possibly captured according to DIA 1979 analytical comments. Last known alive in proximity to enemy forces. (DoD April 1991 list.)

Hunter, Russell P.
USAF–Laos, exited aircraft before crash. (JTF-FA Survival Code 1.)

Huston, Charles G.
USA–Laos, known to be alive on the ground during helicopter exfiltration. When the rope ladder broke and hostile forces approached, the helicopter departed leaving Huston and Brown, alive and unwounded. Search team inserted four days later. No sign of Huston or Brown. (JCRC report.)

Ibanez, Di R.
USMC– Last known alive, DoD April 1991 list.

Jackson, Paul V.
USAF–Laos, known captured according to NSA intercept correlation. (L19, 01D.)

Jakovac, John A.
USA–Believed to have successfully exited his aircraft and was alive on the ground. Last known alive, DoD April 1991 list.

Jewell, Eugene M.
USAF–Hearsay information on possible survival of Jewell obtained by POW returnee Edward Brudo. (Other possibly related hearsay information obtained by POW returnees Risner, Rivers and Rutledge on name "Jual" heard on Voice of Vietnam or camp radio.) Closest correlation is Jewell, Eugene M. USAF.

Johns, Vernon Z.
USA–Hostile capture (DoD June 1973 list). Listed as POW by DIA, 1973. Last seen alive, DIA April 1991 list.

Johnson, Bruce G.
USA–Last known alive, DoD April 1991 list.

Johnson, William D.
USA–Last known alive, DoD April 1991 list.

Johnston, Steven B.

USAF—Laos, exited aircraft before crash. (JTF-FA Survival Code 1.)

Jones, Bobby M.

USAF—POW seen alive in prison camp on November, 1972. (Metzger debrief M133). Hearsay information of Bobby "M" Jones obtained by returnee Mulligan A. "B" Jones was also seen alive in prison by reutrnee Orson G. Swindle.

Finally, POW returnee Richard Vogel also had hearsay information of a POW named Bob Jones. Two beeper signals believed to have been heard following Bobby Jones's incident. (DIA analytical comment.)

Jordon, Larry M.

USN—Crew down and captured in China according to Peking Bulletin and Peking Radio. Information obtained by POW returnee Phillip Smith.

Kennedy, John W.

USAF—Known captured according to NSA intercept correlation.

Ketchie, Scott D.

USMC—Laos, exited aircraft before crash. (JTF-FA Survival Crash Code 2.) Known captured according to NSA intercept correlation.

Kiefel, Ernest P.

USAF—Laos, exited aircraft before crash. (JTF-FA Survival Code 1.)

Kier, Larry G.

USA—Possible POW held in isolation. (S098 debrief-USAF correlation.)

Knutson, Richard A.

USA—POW shot down in January, 1973. Contact and discussion with POW returnee LeBlanc.

Koons, Dale F.

USAF—POW in good physical condition held in the Plantation prison according to firsthand and hearsay reports by returning POWs. (Doss D057, Smith S107, Schwertfeger S182.)

Kosko, Walter

USAF—Military ID card seen in prison. (Berg debrief B083.) Known to have ejected from aircraft.

Kryszak, Theodore E.

USAF—Laos, no trace of crew, wreckage sited.

Kubley, Roy R.

USAF—Laos, survival possible according to DIA 1979 analytical comments.

LaFayette, John W.

USA—Laos, radio contact on ground. (DIA 1979 report.) Exited aircraft before crash. (JTF-FA Survival Code 1.) Believed to have successfully exited his aircraft and was alive on the ground. Last known alive, DoD Alive April 1991 list.

Lane, Charles

USAF—Two good chutes seen. One of the two crew members (unidentified) was known to have been alive on the ground according to Carrigan debrief C078.

Lawrence, Bruce E.

USAF—Name heard in prison system communication according to POW returnee Mulligan M131.

Lee, Leonard M.

USN—Believed to have successfuly exited his aircraft and was alive on the ground. Last known alive, DoD April 1991 list. (DIA 1979 analytical comment.)

Leeser, Leonard C.

USAF—Beeper heard for short period.

Lemon, Jeffrey C.

USAF—Laos, possibly captured alive, according to NSA intercept correlation. (F4D Two-seater, one captured, one found dead.)

Lerner, Irwin S.

USAF—Survived incident, down okay according to crewmember debrief Klomann (K082).

Lester, Roderick B.

USN—Orders given by enemy to capture the two pilots from this aircraft according to NSA intercept correlation.

Lewandowske, Leonard J.

USMC—Name heard on radio and photo seen in magazine according to hearsay information from POW returnee Leo Hyatt.

Lewis, James W.

USAF—Laos, believed to have successfuly exited his aircraft and was alive on the ground. Last known alive, DoD April 1991 list.

Long, John H.

USAF—POW in Hanoi in good physical condition according to firsthand observation by POW returnee Bande. Bande reported Long's full name seen in Citadel, Holiday Inn, Vegas prisons.

Lull, Howard B.

USA—POW, seen alive and evading, and subsequently captured according the POW Returnee Mard Smith and Albert Carlson debriefs.

Luna, Carter P.

USAF—Laos, voice contact on ground. (JTF-FA Survival Code 1.) Listed as POW by DIA in 1973. Likely that he was captured. (DIA 1992 analytical comment.)

Lundy, Albro L.

USAF—Laos, exited aircraft before crash. (JTF-FA Survival Code 1.) Alleged post-capture photo positively identified by family members.

Malone, Jimmy M.

USA—Last known alive, DoD April 1991 list.

Mamiya, John M.

USAF—Identified by Thai returnees, 1973.

Mangino, Charles W.

UAN—Good chute, (DIA report 1979).

Marker, Michael W.
USA—Possibly captured alive according to NSA intercept correlation. (Intercept—three out of five from JU21A incident alive and captured.)

Martin, Russell D.
USAF—Laos, no trace of crew, wreckage found.

Massucci, Martin J.
USAF—Possibly last known alive (one of the two crewmembers were known to have been last known alive—see Scharf, Charles J.) DoD April 1991 list.

Matejoy, Joseph A.
USAF—Laos, EC47Q, Baron 52, believed to have been captured according to analysts in 1973 based on NSA intelligence reports.

Mauterer, Oscar
USAF—Laos, ejected and possibly captured. (DIA analytical comments, 1979 report.) Exited aircraft before crash. (JTF-FA Survival Code 1.) Believed to have successfully gotten out of his aircraft and was alive on the gound. Last known alive, DoD April 1991 list.

McCarty, James L.
USAF—Good chute observed by SAR. (See Jackson J044, Marshall M168, Hanto and McDowell debriefs.) F4D 6/24/72.

McClearly, George C.
USAF—POW later positively identified in 1969 in Christmas photo. (POW returnee Charles C141 and McNish M126 debriefs.)

McCrary, Jack
USAF—Radio contact. (DIA 1979 report.)

McDonald, Joseph W.
USMC—Identified as POW held at Ha Lo prison in good physical condition according to firsthand contact by POW returnee Rayford R049 debrief. "Possibly captured" according to DIA comments, 1979.

McDonald, Kurt C.
USAF—Believed to have successfully gotten out of his aircraft and was alive on the ground. Last known alive, DoD April 1991 list.

McDonnell, John T.
USA—Last known alive, DoD April 1991 list.

McElvain, James R.
USAF—Name possibly heard on radio broadcast. (Shumaker debrief S097.)

McGar, Brian K.
USA—Last known alive, DoD April 1991 list.

McIntire, Scott W.
USAF—Laos, exited aircraft before crash. (JTF-FA Survival Code 1.) Possible POW according to NSA correlation. Possible conflicting SAR information.

McLean, James H.
USA–POW, capture confirmed by Vietnam POWs according to 1979 DIA report. Hostile capture, DoD June 1973 list. Listed as POW by DIA, 1973. Last known alive, DoD April 1991 list.

McPherson, Everett A.
USMC–Name believed to have been passed on prisoner list in Cu Loc prison according to POW returnee Norris Charles debrief.

Mellor, Fredric M.
USAF–Voice contact, uninjured.

Melton, Todd M.
USAF–Laos, EC47Q, Baron 52, believed to have been captured according to analysts in 1973 based on NSA intelligence reports.

Milius, Paul L.
USN–Laos, exited aircraft before crash. (JTF-FA Survival Code 2.)

Millner, Michael
USA–Last known alive, DoD April 1991 list.

Mims, George I.
USAF–Believed to have successfully exited his aircraft before crash and was alive on the ground. (DoD April 1991 list.)

Mitchell, Harry E.
USN–Possibly seen. (1979 DIA report.)

Miyazake, Ronald K.
USAF–Survival possible from crash, but no sign. (According to analytical comments by DIA, 1979.)

Moreland, James L.
USA–Last seen alive and unwounded on the ground according to POW returnee Thompson debrief.

Morgan, James S.
USAF–Believed to have successfully exited his aircraft and was alive on the ground. Last known alive, DoD April 1991 list.

Morris, George W.
USAF–Good chute. Possible voice contact. (Kientzler debrief, DIA 1979 report.) Believed to have successfully exited his aircraft and was alive on the ground. Last known alive, DoD April 1991 list.

Morrissey, Robert D.
USAF–Laos/NVN, Captured alive according to same-day intelligence report indication capture of pilot(s) of a low-flying aircraft in same location and giving orders to "conceal the accomplishment." (No other shootdowns correlate to this report.) Intelligence report one week later requested special Vietnamese team to transport the hulk of an F-111. NSA analyst recalls Brown on list of POWs moved to Sam Neua for movement to USSR. NVN defector states intace portion (possibly the ejection capsule) of an F-111 sent to China same month as Morrissey/Brown shootdown. NVN photographers not allowed to keep photos of F-111.

Monroe, Larry K.
USA—Last known alive, DoD April 1991 list.

Mossman, Harry S.
USN—Orders given by enemy to capture both pilots from this incident according to NSA intercept correlation.

Mullen, William F.
USMC—Laos, exited aircraft before crash. (JTF-FA Survival Code 1.)

Mullins, Harold E.
USAF—Laos, no trace of crew, wreckage sited.

Mundt, Henry G.
USAF—Laos, exited aircraft before crash. (JTF-FA Survival Code 1.) Believed to have successfully exited his aircraft and was alive on the ground. Last known alive, DoD April 1991 list.

Netherland, Roger M.
USN—Believed to have successfully exited his aircraft and was alive on the ground. Last known alive, DoD April 1991 list.

Newton, Charles V.
USA—Last known alive, DoD April 1991 list.

Newton, Donald S.
USA—Last known alive, DoD April 1991 list.

Nichils, Hubert C.
USAF—Name "Nichiles" seen on prison wall at Heartbreak and Zoo prisons in November, 1972. (See POW returnee debriefs Yound Y008, Zuberbuhler Z009 and Brunson B190.) Possible correlation to either Hubert Nicholes or POW returnee Aubrey Nichols.

Nidds, Daniel R.
USA—Last known alive, DoD April 1991 list.

O'Grady, John F.
USAF—Ejected (DIA 1979 report). Captured (NVN sources, 1991.)

Osborne, Rodney L.
USA—Possibly captured alive according to NSA intercept correlation (intercept—three out of five from JU21A incident alive and captured).

Parker, Woodrow, W.
USAF—POW at Citadel and Country Club prisons. Indirect contact (wall tapping) reported by POW returnee Overly (debrief O025).

Parsley, Edward M.
USAF—Reported as possible POW "name familiar." (Coffee debrief C088.)

Paschall, Ronald P.
USA—Pulled alive out of aircraft by crew member prior to explosion. Crew member subsequently captured alone. No further details known. (Astorga debrief.)

Patterson, James Kelly

USN–Alive on ground (four days). (Russell debrief R045.) "Probably captured with broken leg," according to DIA analytical comment, 1979. Hostile capture, DoD June 1973 list. Listed as POW by DIA in 1973. Enemy captors told crew member POW returnee McDaniel that Patterson had been injured but was better now.

Pender, Orland, J.

USN–Possible POW, name heard by returnee Rudloff debrief (R085).

Perrine, Elton L.

USAF–Believed to have succesfully exited his aircraft and was alive on the ground. Last known alive, DoD April 1991 list.

Perry, Randolph A.

USAF–Possibly heard on Voice of Vietnam or camp radio. (Risner, Rivers debriefs.) Name also reported by POW returnees Rutledge and Shumaker.

Peterson, Delbert R.

USAF–Believed to have successfully exited his aircraft and was alive on the ground. Last known alive, DoD April 1991 list.

Peterson, Mark A.

USAF–Good chute. Possible voice contact. (Kientzler debrief, DIA 1979 report.) Believed to have successfully exited his aircraft and was alive on the ground. Last known alive, DoD April 1991 list. Reported as captured according to NSA intercept correlation.

Phillips, Daniel R.

USA–Last seen alive and unwounded during ground fighting by returnee Dennis Thompson.

Phillips, Robert P.

USA–Hostile capture. (DoD June 1973 list.) Listed as POW by DIA, 1973. Last known alive, DoD April 1991 list.

Pierson, William C.

USA–POW according to prison communications and hearsay name on note passed in prison. (Charles and Mulligan POW returnee debriefs.)

Pike, Dennis S.

USN–Laos, exited aircraft before crash.(JTF-FA Survival Code 2.)

Pittmann, Allen D.

USAF–Laos, exited aircraft before crash. (JTF-FA Survival Code 1.)

Plassmeyer, Bernard H.

USMC–Believed to have successfully exited his aircraft and was alive on the ground. Last known alive, DoD April 1991 list.

Platt, Robert L.

USA–Last known alive, DoD April 1991 list.

Plumadore, Kenneth L.

USA–Last known alive, DoD April 1991 list. Captured by PNVA forces (JTF-FA Narrative).

Pogreba, Dean A.
USAF—Believed shot down and captured in China. (Thorsness debrief T03.) Supporting data from Select Committee deposition points toward shoot-down and possible capture of Pogreba in China. Several additional returned POWs reported that Pogreba was believed to have been shot down over China.

Preston, James A.
USAF—Laos, name heard by several returned POWs over Voice of Vietnam or camp radio. (Hyatt, Risner, Rivers, Rutledge Shumaker.)

Prevedel, Charles F.
USA—Last known alive, DoD April 1991 list.

Price, Bunyan D.
USA—Seen alive evading. JSSA list. Helicopter found, no trace of subject. (DIA analytical comment, 1979.) Hostile capture, DoD June 1973 list. Listed as POW by DIA, 1973. Last known alive, DoD April 1991 list.

Pridmore, Dallas R.
USA—Kidnapped from girlfriend's house, South Vietnam (DIA 1979 report). Hostile capture, DoD June 1973 list. Listed as POW by DIA, June 1973. Last known alive, DoD April 1991 list.

Pruett, William D.
USAF—Beeper heard for short period.

Puentes, Manuel F.
USA—Last seen moving, wounded in ambush.

Pugh, Dennis G.
USAF—Laos, exited aircraft before crash. (JTF-FA Survival Code 1.) Known captured according to NSA intercept correlation.

Ransbottom, Frederick J.
USA—POW according to information provided by POW returnee Julius Long. Long had firsthand observation of Ransbottom.

Raymond, Paul D.
USAF—Name heard in prison communication according to POW returnee James Mulligan M131.

Reed, James W.
USAF—Laos, known to have parachuted from aircraft, orders given by enemy to capture the individual according to NSA intercept correlation.

Rehe, Richard R.
USA—Observed wounded at NVA interrogation post in 1968 by POW returnee Daly. Listed as POW by DIA (31 Jan. 92 dep).

Richardson, Dale W.
USA—No trace of subject, helicopter found. (DIA report 1979.) Richardson exited aircraft after it was downed and evaded. (Maslowske, Young and Crowson debriefs.)

Robertson, John L.
USAF–Believed to have successfully exited his aircraft and was alive on the ground. Last known alive, DoD April 1991 list. Positively identified by family members in alleged post-capture photograph.

Roe, Jerry L.
USA–Last known alive, DoD April 1991 list.

Rose, Luther L.
USAF–Laos, no trace of crew, wreckage found.

Ross, Joseph, S.
USAF–Last name seen on prison wall at Heartbreak prison according to Young, Zuberbuhler, and Brunson debriefs. (See Thompson.)

Rowley, Charles S.
USAF–Laos, positively identified as a POW by returnee Lawrence Stark from "either propaganda picture or group of Laos POWs viewing film shown at Hanoi Hilton" with Stark in February, 1973. (Stark debrief.) Additional information obtained from Select Committee deposition of U.S. Embassy official from Laos during war.

Rozo, James Milan
USA–Hostile capture (DoD June 1973 list). Listed as POW by DIA, 1973. Last known alive, DoD April 1991 list.

Russell, Peter, J.
USA–Last known alive, DoD April 1991 list.

Scharf, Charles J.
USAF–Last known alive–one of the two crewmembers were known to have been last known alive (see Massucci, Martin J.), DoD April 1991 list.

Schmidt, Walter R.
USMC–Landed alive, NVA approaching. (DIA 1979 analytical comment.) Captured alive, JSSA. Possibly shot, JSSA. Listed as POW by DIA, 1973. Hostile capture (DoD June 1973 list). Last known alive, DoD April 1991 list.

Schultz, Sheldon D.
USA–Laos, no sign of crew.

Schumann, John R.
USA–POW last known alive working on a rice mill, heavy manual labor, chopping wood, 40 push-ups, developed congested lungs according to POW returnee Douglas Ramsey.

Scull, Gary B.
USA–Last known alive, DoD April 1991 list. NSA correlation March 13, 1970.

Serex, Henry M.
USAF–Possibly survived as prisoner of war. (Information under Committee evaluation–one person from crew known captured according to NSA intercept correlation.)

Seymore, Leo E.
USA–Laos, last known alive, DoD April 1991 list.

Shafer, Phillip R.

USA—Listed as POW by DIA, 1973. Last known alive, DoD April 1991 list. Possible propaganda broadcast made by Shafer while in captivity.

Shark, Earl E.

USA—Listed as POW by DoD PW/MIA Task Group.

Shelton, Charles

USAF—Captured by Pathet Lao forces, voice contact.

Shinn, William C.

USAF—Beeper heard for short period.

Shriver, Jerry M.

USA—POW according to POW returnee Norris Charles. "Charles seems positive this man is a POW," (USAF 1973 comment).

Sigafoos, Walter H.

USAF—Laos, possibly captured according to NSA intercept correlation (F4D two-seater, one captured, one found dead).

Singleton, Daniel L

USAF—Laos, possibly captured according to NSA intercept correlation. (F4E-two-seater—one captured.) POW early returnee (1969) Wesley Rumble listed a "Larry Singleton" on a list of hearsay names that he was given to memorize. Singleton was shot down in January, 1969.

Sittner, Ronald N.

USAF—Two good chutes seen. One of the two crewmembers (unidentified) was known to have been alive on the ground according to Carrigan debrief C078.

Skinner, Owen G.

USAF—Laos, exited aircraft before crash. (JTF-FA Survival Code 1.)

Small, Burt C.

USA—Captured with wounded leg. DIA 1979 report. Listed as POW by DIA, 1973. Hostile capture, DoD June 1973 report. Last known alive, DoD April 1991 list.

Smith, Harding E.

USAF—Laos, no trace of crew, wreckage found.

Smith, Warren P.

USAF—Laos, exited aircraft before crash. (JTF-FA Survival Code 1.)

Soyland, David P.

USA—Last known alive, DoD April 1991 list.

Sparks, Donald L.

USA—Sent letter home as POW. Last seen with wounded foot. (JSSA list, DIA 1979.) Listed as POW by DIA, 1973. Hostile capture (DoD June 1973 list). Last known alive, DoD April 1991 list. Known to have been captured according to several returnees. Firsthand observation claimed by POW returnee Carroll Flora on March 5, 1973 at Ha Lo, Vegas, Hanoi Hilton prisons.

Sparks, Jon M.

USA—Laos, exited aircraft before crash. (JTF-FA Survival Code 1.)

Spinelli, Domenick A.

USN–Possible POW. Name referenced by POW returnee Richard George Tangeman. Spinelli subject of subsequent post-war live-sighting information.

Steen, Martin W.

USAF–Good chute (DIA 1979). Possibly alive when found. (Young debrief.)

Stevens, Larry J.

USN–Laos, alleged post-capture photograph positively identified by family members.

Stewart, Peter J.

USAF–Alleged post-capture photograph positively identified by family member.

Steware, Virgil, G.

USAF–Laos, exited aircraft before crash. (JTF-FA Survival Code 1.)

Strait, Douglas F.

USA–Believed to have successfully exited aircraft (OH6A) and was alive on the ground. Last known alive, DoD April 1991 list.

Strawn, John T.

USA–Possibly captured alive according to NSA intercept correlation. (Intercept-three out of five from JU21A incident alive and captured.)

Strohlein, Madison A.

USA–Last known alive, DoD April 1991 list.

Sutton, Wiliam C.

USAF–Beeper heard for short period.

Tatum, Lawrence B.

USAF–Believed to have successfully exited his aircraft and was alive on the ground. Last known alive, DoD April 1991 list.

Taylor, Fred

USA–Last known alive, DoD April 1991 list.

Thompson, William J.

USAF–POW according to secondhand report of wall-tapping. (Vohden debrief.) Secondhand information from CIA captive Weaver. (See Ross.)

Tigner, Lee M.

USAF–Possibly captured according to NSA intercept correlation. (One pilot captured from two-seater aircraft.)

Townsend, Francis W.

USAF–Listed as POW by DIA, 1973. Last known alive, DoD April 1991 list. Known to have ejected from aircraft (POW returnee Gauntt debrief).

Trent, Alan R.

USAF–Cambodia, possibly captured according to NSA intercept correlation. (F4D two-seater, one pilot captured.)

Tromp, William L.

USN–Hostile capture (DoD June 1973 list). Listed as POW by DIA 1973. Last known alive, DoD April 1991 list.

Utley, Russel K.
USAF—Laos, possibly captured according to NSA intercept correlation. (F4E two-seater, one captured.)

Walker, Bruce C.
USAF—Believed to have successfully exited his aircraft and was alive on the ground. Last known alive, DoD April 1991 list. Known to have evaded for 11 days, maintaining radio contact. (DIA 1979 analytical comment). Spotter aircraft subsequently reported Walker was surrounded by 40 NVA troops. Known captured according to NSA intercept correlation. Military ID card found in Hanoi military museum (January, 1992).

Walker, Lloyd F.
USAF—Laos, survival possible but no sign. (DIA 1979 analytical comments.)

Walker, Samuel F.
USAF—Laos, one parachute observed, mid-air collision. (DIA analytical comment 1979.)

Walton, Lewis C.
USA—Radio interception indicated Walton and Entrican had been captured and were to be moved north to Hanoi according to POW returnee. (See returnee debrief Jon Cavaiani C139.) Note: DIA suspects Entrican was captured by hostile forces. Entrican and Walton were together.

Warren, Gray D.
USAF—Laos, no trace of crew, wreckage found. (DIA analytical comment, 1979.)

Wheeler, Eugene L.
USMC—Voice contact, last known alive, DoD April 1991 list.

White, Charles E.
USA—Last known alive, DoD April 1991 list.

Wilkins, George H.
USN—Identified alive by Thai returnees.

Williams, Robert J.
USA—POW reportedly seen in Vietnamese magazine photograph, JSSA.

Williamson, James D.
USA—Laos, POW according to hearsay information, JSSA. No sign of crew, DIA. Believed by POW returnee Friese and Uyeyama to have signed propaganda statement.

Winters, David M.
USA—Last known alive, DoD April 1991 list.

Worth, James F.
USMC—Last known alive, DoD April 1991 list.

Wood, Don C.
USAF—Laos, identified in Pathet Lao film, possibly captured. (DIA, 1979.) Believed to have successfully exited his aircraft and was alive on the ground. Last known alive, DOD April 1991 list.

Wood, William C.
USAF—Laos, exited aircraft before crash. (JTF-FA Survival Code 1.)

Wright, David I.

USAF–Possibly captured according to NSA intercept correlation. (One captured from crew of two.)

Wright, Thomas T.

USAF–Laos, believed to have successfully exited his aircraft and was alive on the ground. Last known alive, DoD April 1991 list.

Wrobleske, Walter F.

USA–Last known alive, DoD April 1991 list.

Zich, Larry A.

USA–POW seen alive in early 1973 according to POW returnee Lawrence Stark. Zich was believed to be among a group of POWs viewing a propaganda film in late February/early March according to Stark, or had been seen in a propaganda photograph.

Part 5

Be not far from me, for trouble is near,
and there is none to help.

Psalms 22:11

General Overview on POW/MIAs

The Indochina War

According to the Department of Defense, with the signing of the Paris Peace Accords in 1973, America believed it had established the mechanism to achieve a full accounting of American servicemen and civilians still listed as missing from the war in Southeast Asia. However, in April 1973 at the completion of **"Operation Homecoming,"** the repatriation of our POWs, only 591 had returned.

Many more remained unaccounted for and it became obvious that the Paris Agreement would not be honored. Despite the efforts of government agencies, families of POW/MIAs, and private organizations, throughout the years since the Paris Agreements, the governments of Indochina failed to provide the answers that continue to keep this issue on the minds of the American people.

Since 1973, continuous diplomatic contacts with the Indochinese governments have slowly but positively improved the level of cooperation received in our search for answers. Today, our success can be measured in quantifiable terms.

We have formalized a short-notice live-sighting system where our investigators can rapidly respond to reports of sightings of live Americans in these countries. We conduct multiple joint field activities with the Southeast Asian governments where we are on the ground investigating and excavating crash sites and grave sites of missing Americans.

Also, there is an important fact of the 318 U.S. remains returned and identified since 1973. To improve on these successes, we continue to press for access to historical wartime records and archives, a source undoubtedly rich with information relevant to the fates of our people. Our efforts are beginning to bear fruit. Recently, the Vietnamese government has finally committed to provide our investigators access to these records and archives.

The U.S. government policy is to investigate each and every case in the pursuit of the fullest possible accounting of the missing. Since the possibility that some MIAs may still be alive cannot be eliminated, U.S. negotiators have identified a representative sampling of "discrepancy" cases where the best opportunity for survival indicates the Vietnamese government should be able to provide immediate answers.

These 135 cases, commonly referred to as the "compelling" or "discrepancy" cases, are ones in which the preponderance of information indicates that these individuals survived their incident of loss and were either captured by, killed by or located in the proximity of enemy forces.

In any case, the government of Hanoi should be able to provide a great deal of information concerning these individuals or lead us to their remains. The particulars of these cases have been repeatedly presented to the Vietnamese who agreed to the completion of the investigation of the discrepancy cases by January 1993.

World War II, Korean War, and the Cold War

Following World War II, the U.S. government, together with our Allies around the world, engaged in a concerted effort to return liberated Prisoners of War to their respective homelands, identify and repatriate remains of fallen servicemen, and pay proper respect to those servicemen who could not be identified. As the Soviet government became more adversarial, access to information on American servicemen in Soviet control became nonexistent.

In Korea, the pattern was repeated. Large numbers of U.S. servicemen were reported missing following combat operations involving North Korean and Communist Chinese forces. Over 8,100 of these individuals were never accounted for, and efforts by the United Nations to obtain an accurate accounting have been less than successful.

Throughout the Cold War, U.S. reconnaissance aircraft, flying along the borders of Communist-controlled territory, have on occasion been engaged by Communist forces. In addition, U.S. servicemen and civilians have been the subject of kidnapings in areas like West Berlin, where individuals were in close proximity to Soviet-controlled territory. Diplomatic efforts to secure the release of individuals involved in these circumstances have met with limited success.

U.S. government efforts in the past to account for American servicemen from World War II, the Korean War and the Cold War have been restricted due to the lack of cooperation by Communist governments. The collapse of the former Soviet Union has afforded us with the opportunity to address many of these questions with renewed vigor.

The Department of Defense has taken the lead role in the work of the U.S.–Russian Joint Commission on POW/MIAs. The objectives of this bilateral Commission include pursuing information that will lead to an accounting of missing servicemen from WWII, Korea and the Cold

War. Through the Joint Commission, the U.S. government will pursue every lead and investigate every source of information to obtain as complete an accounting as possible of our fellow countrymen.

Outside the U.S.–Russian Joint Commission, the U.S. government continues to query the government of the Peoples Republic of China and North Korea for any information that could assist in accounting of servicemen who may have been lost during the Korean War and the Cold War. We will continue to pursue every avenue available to the Department of Defense to secure greater cooperation with these two countries.

Operation Desert Storm

Operation Desert Storm was completed with a full accounting of the American participants. Although several factors contributed to the success of this operation, such as desert terrain and improved communications equipment, what we learned from the experiences of the past were clearly the catalyst that helped to improve the overall effort.

Future Conflicts

The Department of Defense is committed to upgrading systems and procedures that will provide for the total accounting of U.S. personnel during times of conflict. Building on the foundation of past experiences, we have clarified and streamlined areas of responsibilities. We continue to strive to provide the agencies responsible for these activities with the best equipment available to perform their tasks. We are beginning to incorporate new medical technologies, such as DNA typing, that will significantly enhance our ability to identify casualties. In the event that the United States is forced into armed conflict in the future, the Department of Defense stands ready.

Summary

Today the search continues with a new intensity. With the reaffirmation of commitment from the President and Secretary Cheney, significant resources from across the U.S. government have been applied to this effort.

Americans Unaccounted For In Southeast Asia.

Following the return of the American prisoners of war during Operation Homecoming in 1973, there were 1,259 Americans still listed as missing and 1,124 Americans listed as killed in action whose remains had not been recovered.

This latter group was referred to KIA/BNR. The missing Americans were further categorized as either POW/MIA based upon the known circumstances surrounding the individual's loss at the time of the incident. By the early 1980s administrative reviews, under the provisions of Title 37

U.S. Code (The Missing Persons Act), were conducted for each incident involving a missing American.

The law directed that a review of each incident be conducted and, based upon existing evidence, either continue the individual in a missing status or make a finding of death. A finding of death could be based on either a presumptive finding that the individual could not have survived or conclusive evidence that the individual had died.

As a result of these reviews, findings of death were rendered in each case and the individuals were subsequently listed as KIA/BNR with the exception of one individual. That individual is still categorized as captured and listed as a prisoner of war to symbolize the Administrations's commitment to the fullest possible accounting of all our personnel from the conflict in Southeast Asia.

A finding of death is required by law and is made for administrative and legal purposes only. It does not change the way the U.S. government proceeds to account for missing service personnel and civilians. The U.S. government operates under the assumption that some missing men could still be alive.

Listing Of Remaining Unresolved U.S. Losses By Service Component

Component	POW/MIA*	KIA/MIA*	TOTAL
Army	356	316	673
Navy	120	328	448
Marine Corps	104	179	283
Air Force	553	265	818
Coast Guard	0	1	1
Civilian	37	5	42
TOTAL	****1170**	**1094**	**2265**

*Original categories existing at the conclusion of hostilities in January 1973.

**As a result of actions taken by administrative review boards convened under the provision of Title 37 of the U.S. Code, these cases were changed from their original status of "Captured" or "Missing" to KIA/BNR in the early 1980s. All unaccounted for Americans from the Indochina War are officially listed as KIA/BNR with the exception of one case (Shelton) who is still carried as "Captured" as a symbolic gesture.

As of October 15, 1992, there were 2,265 Americans still missing and unaccounted for as a result of U.S. involvement in the conflict in Southeast Asia. A breakdown by country of loss follows:

Americans Unaccounted For In Southeast Asia

Country Of Loss	Total
North Vietnam	604
South Vietnam	1,053
Laos	519
Cambodia	81
China	8
TOTAL	**2,265**

U.S. Servicemen Unaccounted For By State

Alabama—42	Nebraska—21
Alaska—2	Nevada—8
Arizona—23	New Hampshire—10
Arkansas—26	New Jersey—59
California—227	New Mexico—17
Colorado—39	New York—144
Connecticut—37	North Carolina—55
Delaware—5	North Dakota—16
District of Columbia— 9	Ohio—112
Florida—77	Oklahoma—47
Georgia—43	Oregon—43
Hawaii—10	Pennsylvania—113
Idaho—11	Rhode Island—9
Illinois—94	South Carolina—30
Indiana—65	South Dakota—8
Iowa—38	Tennessee—42
Kansas—35	Texas—145
Kentucky—21	Utah—19
Louisiana—29	Vermont—4
Maine—17	Virginia—54
Maryland—35	Washington—55
Massachusetts—54	West Virginia—23
Michigan—72	Wisconsin—37
Minnesota—41	Wyoming—6
Mississippi—18	Puerto Rico—2
Missouri—48	Virgin Islands—1
Montana—20	Other—7

Note: Does not include 42 civilians

The Indochinese Governments Hold The Answers

The U. S. government has consistently urged senior officials in the three Indochinese countries to meet their humanitarian obligation to provide the fullest possible accounting of missing Americans. While these governments assert that they hold no live Americans and have increased cooperation on accounting efforts, it is clear that considerably more information on, and remains of, missing Americans could be provided, particularly by Vietnam.

As a matter of highest national priority, the United States is committed to repatriating any Americans who may still be held captive, obtaining the fullest possible accounting for Americans still missing in Southeast Asia and returning all recoverable remains.

Socialist Republic Of Vietnam (SRV)

There is convincing evidence that the Vietnamese government has knowledge concerning hundreds of U.S. servicemen lost in Vietnam, especially over the northern part of the country and in areas of Laos and Cambodia which were under the control of Vietnamese forces during the war.

For instance, thoughout the war a wealth of information on specific U.S. aircraft loss incidents was published by Vietnam's government-controlled media. Further, public security, militia and regular military units established an effective nationwide ability to capture and process prisoners of war, investigate crashed aircraft, bury remains and report incidents to central authorities.

Burial of an American prisoner, whether in the North or South, was to be reported to Hanoi as quickly as possible along with sketches of the burial site. In 1978, a Vietnamese mortician provided the U.S. with credible information on over 400 American remains which were then stored in Hanoi. Since that time, only 268 remains have been returned and identified, 60 percent with evidence of storage.

Lao Peoples Democratic Republic (LPDR)

As part of "Operation Homecoming" in early 1973, nine U.S. servicemen who had been captured in Laos were released in Hanoi. These men had not been captured by the Pathet Lao, but by Vietnamese soldier operations in Laos. Later in 1973, a peace agreement was signed between the Royal Lao government and Pathet Lao forces.

While the United States was not a signatory, the agreement specified conditions and provisions for the exchange of prisoners of war, regardless of nationality, and information on the missing. Publicly, the Pathet Lao had often stated that they held scores of Americans. After signing the agreement, they claimed to hold only U.S. civilian pilot Emmet Kay, captured on May 7, 1973, and that the Central Committee had been gathering information on missing U.S. personnel, but cautioned that they could probably provide information on only a "feeble percentage."

In 1978, the Lao Government provided the remains of four persons to a visiting congressional delegation. Two of the remains were determined to be those of indigenous Southeast Asians. One of the remaining two was identified as a USAF pilot whose plane was shot down on the Lao/Vietnam border; the forth set of remains is still inidentified. Since 1973, 43 Americans previously missing in Laos have been accounted for as a result of joint U.S./Lao efforts.

The small number of Americans accounted for in Laos can, in part, be explained by the fact that the majority of the 519 unresolved American losses occurred in areas then under near-total control by Vietnamese forces. These losses were primarily in eastern Laos, along the Vietnam border and the Ho Chi Minh Trail complex.

The U.S. government believes that the Vietnamese government has records on these incidents which could help account for many of these men. At U.S. urging, both the Vietnamese and Lao have agreed in principle to cooperate trilaterally with us in an effort to resolve these cases. The Lao government should, however, be able to account for a number of individuals about whom there is strong evidence of capture by Pathet Lao. Such cases are prioritized for joint investigation.

State Of Cambodia

In Eastern Cambodia where most missing Americans were lost, Vietnamese forces' presence and control were similar to that in Eastern Laos. Most incidents involving U.S. personnel occurred in contact with Vietnamese forces. Vietnamese military records and reports should contain information on these Americans.

It is doubtful that the current leadership in Phnom Penh can provide a significant accounting for Americans missing in Cambodia unless information in the possession of the U.S. and the other Indochina governments is provided to them. Information on a small number of American civilians, including journalists, who reportedly died at the hands of the Khmer Rouge, may appear in records of that era.

Are Americans Still Held Captive In Indochina?

Only the Vietnamese, Lao and the Cambodians know the answer. Nevertheless, taking into consideration the incident circumstances of some Americans, to include last known alive discrepancy cases, and unresolved live-sighting reports, the U.S. government operates on the assumption that some are still alive.

This position is bolstered by the failure of the Indochinese governments, particularly Vietnam, to provide clarifying information or remains which could account for these individuals.

Current United States Government Policy

Although we have thus far been unable to prove that Americans are still detained against their will, the information available to us precludes ruling out that possibility.

Actions to investigate live-sighting reports receive and will continue to receive necessary priority and resources based on the assumption that at least some Americans are still held captive. Should any report prove true, we will take appropriate action to ensure the return of those involved.

The Political Environment

Efforts to account for Americans missing from the Vietnam War have varied in their success depending upon a variety of reasons that include the priority placed on the issue by the U.S. government, the international political situation at the time and Vietnam's perception of its self-interest in responding to these and internal political developments.

Success in accounting for all U.S. personnel missing in Vietnam, as well as a majority of those missing in Laos and Cambodia, depends primarily upon Vietnam's seriousness in cooperation and implementing agreements. For this reason, the following brief chronology describes the political environment affecting the level of Vietnamese cooperation on the POW/MIA issue:

1976–1978: After the end of the war, Vietnam's objective was to be accepted in international fora, such as the United Nations. For example, in 1977 when the U.S. opted not to veto their UN membership, the Vietnamese responded by suddenly repatriating the remains of more than 20 Americans. At the same time, U.S.–Vietnamese negotiations were exploring the possibility of normalizing relations; however, this was later scuttled by Vietnamese demands for war reparations and their invasion of Cambodia. U.S. policy at the time was that the accounting of missing Americans was "a hoped for by-product" of the normalization process.

1978–1982: Following the breakdown of normalization talks, contact with Vietnamese officials virtually halted, as did the return of remains and any form of cooperation on the POW/MIA issue.

1982–Present: The U.S. made clear that resolution of the POW/MIA issue was a humanitarian matter that rested on the international standards and that it was in Vietnam's interest to treat it that way, regardless of the state of U.S./SRV diplomatic relations.

It was also made clear that the U.S. domestic environment, absent such treatment, would dictate that the pace and scope of U.S./SRV relations would be directly affected by cooperation on this issue.

In April 1991, this policy was clarified by the establishment of a "road map" of quid pro quo concrete steps that could be taken by the U.S. in response to SRV cooperation on POW/MIA and Cambodia settlement-related issues. These steps were designed to enhance the pace and scope of our overall relationship.

In response to Vietnamese agreements in October 1991 to increase co-operation on POW/MIA matters and increase access provided to U.S. investigators throughout Indochina, Cheney activated Joint Task Force-Full Accounting within the United States Pacific Command in January 1992. This Joint Task Force enables the U.S. government to focus the vast military resources of the Pacific Command on in-country operations to facilitate achieving the fullest possible accounting for Americans missing in Indochina.

Strengthened Vietnamese agreements reached in March 1992 prompted policy officials in Washington to lift certain aspects of the trade embargo with Vietnam including the ban on telecommunications and two other humanitarian-related steps. The first was to grant an exception to the economic embargo with Vietnam to permit commercial sales to meet basic human needs. The second was to lift restrictions on projects by non-governmental and non-profit organizations in Vietnam.

The Department of Defense is firmly committed to the "road map" policy which provides assurances that U.S. POW/MIA objectives are met and balances the many other humanitarian, economic, legal and diplomatic interests in a series of confidence-building steps leading to normal relations. The key to further steps to improve relations with Vietnam is full implementation of bilateral agreements and POW/MIA results.

Laos

The United States maintained diplomatic relations with Laos throughout the war and to the present. Since 1982, U.S. policy has been to upgrade the bilateral relationship; the principle measure of Lao sincerity in that process was to be their cooperation to resolve the POW/MIA issue.

This policy was amended in 1985 to include steps to counter production and trafficking of narcotics. Since the initial stages, the Lao government has improved the level of POW/MIA and counter-narcotics actions, and the U.S. has sought to respond by providing humanitarian assistance to the Lao people within legal and policy constraints.

The United States and Laos upgraded their relations in July 1992 by establishing full ambassadorial posts in both countries. The President named Charles B. Salmon, Jr., as U.S. Ambassador to Laos, the first U.S. Ambassador since 1975.

The Lao have agreed to an increased tempo of joint field operations over the past two years. Implementation of their 1992 agreements has brought five joint field operations. While the pace of activities has increased significantly over the past eight months, greater flexibility and more time in the field are necessary to gain more rapid results. Hopefully, the Lao government's cooperation on POW/MIA operations will continue to improve.

Cambodia

Over the past year, the U.S. government has made important inroads in POW/MIA cooperation in Cambodia. During July 1991, U.S. POW/MIA investigators traveled to Phnom Penh to investigate a number of photographs purported to depict Americans in captivity. The cooperation of the Cambodian government was instrumental in the successful conclusion of those investigations.

After the signing of the comprehensive political settlement agreement in Paris in October 1991, investigation and recovery teams from Joint Task Force-Full Accounting and the CIL-HI undertook several joint operations with Cambodia counterparts, recovering remains with the Mayaguez incident, and more recently, remains associated with last known alive cases of missing American journalists.

Cambodian cooperation on the POW/MIA issue has been outstanding. In addition to unprecedented access to prisons and other sites of investigative interest, the Cambodians have agreed to the use of U.S. government helicopters, flown by U.S. pilots, for joint field activities. This has enabled U.S. teams to increase flexibility during operations and dramatically improve the safety of U.S. team members on helicopter operations.

U.S. Remains Returned After 1973

Year	Vietnam	Laos
1974	23	0
1975	3	0
1976	2	0
1977	33	0
1978	11	1
1979	0	0
1980	0	1
1981	3	0
1982	4	1
1983	8	1
1984	6	0
1985	38	13
1986	13	9
1987	8	0
1988	62	1
1989	34	7
1990	17	7
1991	4	6
1992	0	0
TOTAL	**269**	**47**

U.S. Government Efforts To Obtain
the Fullest Possible Accounting

The United States government has significantly increased the scope of its efforts on the POW/MIA investigations. Within the Department of Defense alone they have seen a threefold increase in assets and personnel assigned to this task.

In November 1991, Secreatary Cheney established the office of the Deputy Assistant Secretary of Defense (DASD) for POW/MIA Affairs. This represented the first time a DSAD-level position had been assigned to handle a single issue such as POW/MIA and focused the full influence of the highest levels of government on this important effort. In January 1992, Mr. Alan C. Atak was appointed to the new position and was authorized a staff of 14 to orchestrate DoD-wide efforts to find the answers to this longtime problem.

Also in January 1992, the 150-member JTF-FA was established. This joint task force was designed to combine all the specialties necessary to conduct the wide range of operations necessary to obtain the fullest possible accounting goal of the U.S. government. The JTF was placed within the organization of the Commander-in-Chief, United States Pacific Command (USCINCPAC) in Hawaii to allow the full resources of this theater commander to be brought to bear on this effort.

Current United States government policy regarding the POW/MIA issue is coordinated through the POW/MIA IAG. Membership in the IAG includes the Defense Department, the White House National Security Council (NSC) staff, the State Department, the Joint Chiefs of Staff (JCS) and the National League of Families of American Prisoners and Missing in Southeast Asia.

The DIA's Special Office for POW/MIAs serves as the non-voting intelligence representative and adviser to the IAG. The IAG develops integrated policy to resolve the POW/MIA issue, monitors implementation and assesses current efforts, while evaluating new initiatives and approaches. What follows is a historical profile of the United States government efforts in Southeast Asia.

Vietnam

Wartime and post-conflict recovery efforts were the responsibility of the Joint Personnel Recovery Center (JPRC) activated on September 17, 1966 as an integral part of the Military Assistance Command, Vietnam-Special Operations Group.

The Joint Personnel Recovery Center provided an operational focal point and enabled U.S. forces to capitalize on the intelligence network in place at the time. Operationally, its purpose was to plan, coordinate and, in some cases, direct the recovery of American evadees or prisoners. In addition, they had the long-term task of recovering U.S. personnel after search and rescue operations had been suspended.

JPRC agents and operatives were authorized to deal directly with neutral parties or enemy personnel willing to provide information on prisoners for a monetary award or favorable consideration by U.S./Republic of Vietnam authorities.

This information included live-sighting reports, known and suspected POW camp locations, rallier and agent reports, and debriefings of escapees and returnees. The most significant intelligence information was compiled into dossiers on individual cases and multiple losses. This system, code named "Bright Light," would eventually be computerized for instant search and information retrieval and serve to form the basis of the database of information used today.

By the time that U.S. ground combat would formally cease, the JPRC had formed the nucleus of an organization that would become an instrument of the Paris Peace Accords.

Most Americans felt that with the signing of the agreements ending the war in Indochina, accounting for our missing countrymen would finally begin. The then Democratic Republic of Vietnam (DRV), North Vietnam, was expected to honor Article 8 of the Paris Agreement which specifically provided for repatriating POWs from all sides, as well as exchanging information about the missing and returning the remains of those who had died.

These points were conditional only on the withdrawal of U.S. and allied forces from Vietnam. The agreement ending the war in Laos had less specific articles which pertained to repatriating and accounting for POWs and MIAs of all nationalities.

To implement Article 8, the Four Party Joint Military Team (FPJMT) was established. Prior to the fall of the Republic of Vietnam in 1975, under the auspices of the FPJMT, numerous meetings were held where the U.S. negotiators continually pressed for information on the missing.

During the same period, despite the lack of cooperation from the Vietnamese, the Joint Casualty Resolution Center (JCRC), formerly the JPRC, augmented by members from the U.S. Army CIL, Thailand, and other units, were able to conduct limited searches.

These efforts ceased in December 1973 when a search party visiting a pre-announced site was ambushed by Communist forces and an American was killed. During March 1974, North Vietnam returned the remains of 23 U.S. servicemen who had died in captivity.

In the first six years after the fall of the Republic of Vietnam, U.S. Government officials had intermittent and largely unproductive contacts with the Vietnamese on this issue. The House of Representatives established the Select Committee on Missing Persons in Southeast Asia which, during its 15-month tenure (1975-1976), had several contacts with the Vietnamese in Hanoi, Paris, and the United Nations.

In 1977, President Carter appointed Leonard Woodcock to head a Presidential commission on Americans Missing and Unaccounted for in Southeast Asia. This commission visited both Vietnam and Laos to discuss the POW/MIA issue. It was during their March 1977 visit that the Vietnamese first announced that they had established an office to seek information on missing Americans and recover remains.

In addition, Vietnamese officials visited the JCRC and CIL at its new location in Hawaii in July 1978; technical-level meetings were held in Hanoi in October 1980 and May 1981.

Stepped Up Efforts

In 1981, President Reagan established resolution of the POW/MIA issue a matter of the highest national priority, a position strongly reaffirmed by President Bush. The United States government has used all available diplomatic opportunities to persuade the governments of Vietnam and Laos, as well as officials in Cambodia, to cooperate fully on this humanitarian issue.

In addition to emphasizing the humanitarian nature of this problem, the U.S government stressed that resolving the POW/MIA issue in a timely and comprehensive manner was in the best interest of the U.S. and the Indochinese countries.

Progress has been painfully slow, punctuated by periods of cooperation and halts, primarily due to Vietnamese attempts to manipulate the issue for their political advantage.

Over the past 10 years, senior U.S. officials have met with Socialist Republic of Vietnam (SRV) officials on countless occasions attempting to establish the necessary level of cooperation on the POW/MIA issue and other urgent humanitarian concerns.

In addition, regular technical-level meetings were held, and joint field operations have been conducted. Throughout these years, the Vietnamese promised more than they delivered. Despite specific agreements, the Vietnamese often tied pledges of POW/MIA cooperation to political questions.

Whether this pattern was due to internal political differences or a calculated strategy to exploit this issue in a mistaken belief that U.S. concessions on political questions would be possible, the result was the same—

raised hopes of the American people and the POW/MIA families were dashed.

Each policy or technical meeting was important in its own right and helped to increase communications and understanding of expectations. The meetings described below were key in furthering the effort.

In February 1982, a U.S. policy-level delegation held talks in Hanoi which resulted in SRV agreement to hold four technical meetings a year between the U.S. JCRC/CIL-HI and the Vietnamese Office for Seeking Missing Personnel (VNOSMO). The first meeting was not held until December 1982, the second in March 1983, and a third in June 1983. The Vietnamese then interrupted the schedule.

In October 1983, White House and National League of Families Officials met in New York with Vietnamese Foreign Minister Nguyen Co Thack. Discussions focused on overcoming obstacles to advance serious, high-level negotiations between the two governments and lay the groundwork for future cooperation.

A policy-level delegation, led by Assistant Secretary of Defense for International Security Affairs and comprised of officials from the White House, League of Families, State and Defense, traveled to Hanoi in February 1984. Agreement was reached to accelerate cooperation and de-link the POW/MIA issue from U.S.–Vietnamese relations in other areas.

Hanoi also agreed to focus initial efforts on the "most accessible cases in the Hanoi/Haiphong area" and those listed as having died in captivity in southern Vietnam. A technical meeting was subsequently held in August.

In October, U.S. government and League of Families representatives met again with Minister Thack in New York. He renewed and strengthened the February commitments and agreed to set an early date for the next technical meeting held later that month in Vietnam.

Following a March 1985 policy-level delegation visit to Hanoi, a delegation in August, led by a member of the White House staff, returned to discuss Hanoi's newly-announced agreement to resolve the POW/MIA issue within two years. Prior to the delegation's arrival, the U.S. presented a proposed joint plan to accomplish that objective, which would have concluded with nationwide joint investigations of live-sighting reports, surveys and excavations of suspected loss locations.

The U.S. plan also provided an extensive list of U.S. supporting actions. Vietnamese officials did not react to the joint plan but provided their own plan and requested U.S. reaction. In September, a follow-up meeting was held in New York at which time the U.S. provided comments on Vietnam's two-year work plan.

The SRV agreed for the first time to a joint crash site excavation, which occurred in November 1985. In addition, six technical meetings took place that year and Vietnamese unilateral repatriations of remains dramatically expanded. In 1985, 38 remains were repatriated in comparison to only six the year before.

In January 1986, a high-level U.S. government delegation went to Hanoi where senior Vietnamese officials reaffirmed that the POW/MIA issue is a humanitarian one and reiterated their pledge to resolve the issue within two years. They also agreed to investigate any POW live-sighting information that the U.S. might present.

While a technical meeting took place in Hanoi in February, the Vietnamese postponed the planned April meeting to protest the U.S. government retaliatory actions against Libya to counter international terrorism. The delayed technical talks, finally held in June, merely provided a forum for ongoing Vietnamese criticism of the U.S. for not fulfilling its commitments to the Vietnamese plan.

A May 1986 policy-level meeting with the Vietnamese in New York was followed by a June technical meeting and a White House led Interagency delegation to Hanoi in July. This group met with Minister Thack to formalize U.S. commitments to support Vietnam's unilateral two-year plan, but rejected any political linkage.

The meeting also resulted in agreements that technical talks would be held in August and October; that at least six such meetings would be held per year; that U.S. and the SRV forensic specialists would consult in Vietnam; and that the SRV would provide the U.S. with written results of its investigations into reports of live-sightings. Moreover, the SRV agreed to permit U.S. experts to accompany its officials on investigations in accessible areas, discuss specific crash sites for excavation and accepted an invitation to visit the U.S. technical facilities at the JCRC and CIL-HI. While the August and October technical meetings did take place, the Vietnamese publicly began to back away from some of their commitments.

In January 1987, U.S. proposals for technical discussions in Hanoi were rejected by the Vietnamese, as was a similar proposal the following month. In an effort to increase momentum for resolving this pressing humanitarian issue, President Reagan named General Vessey, as Special Presidential Emissary to Hanoi for POW/MIA Affairs. Following difficult negotiations to establish an agreed upon agenda, General Vessey led an Interagency Group delegation to Hanoi in August 1987.

During these meetings, General Vessey obtained agreement to resume and expand cooperation on POW/MIA and other humanitarian issues of mutual concern. The two sides reaffirmed the need to focus first on discrepancy cases and on Americans listed as having died in captivity in South Vietnam. Representative case files were provided for Vietnamese considerations. General Vessey also indicated that the U.S. could not consider direct aid to Vietnam due to existing law but would address within policy and legal constraints certain humanitarian concerns of the Vietnamese people, specifically by encouraging American non-governmental organizations to provide prosthetics assistance to Vietnam's disabled. This was later expanded to encompass child health and survival assistance.

General Vessey continued to maintain contact with Vietnamese officials and in September 1987 led a delegation to New York for a meeting with Vietnam's Vice Foreign Minister to discuss the progress on commitments made the previous month. Two technical meetings in Hanoi, between U.S. Representatives and their Vietnamese counterparts also took place before the end of 1987.

In 1988, Vietnam agreed to initiate joint field investigations aimed at resolving "compelling" cases that General Vessey had previously provided and to expand their unilateral efforts. This agreement in principle was reached during a June meeting in New York between a U.S. Delegation led by General Vessey and Minister Thach.

It was followed by a Vietnamese return visit to the JCRC and CIL-HI where they were briefed on technical and forensic capabilities to enhance the accounting effort.

During the July technical meeting in Hanoi, the Vietnamese presented proposals for the joint activities and, at a subsequent meeting, agreed to begin the joint investigations on September 25.

In all, six technical talks on the POW/MIA issue were held in 1988 and unilateral remains repatriations by Vietnam again significantly increased. In 1988 the Vietnamese repatriated 62 sets of remains while they had only returned eight in 1987.

A separate U.S. team continued to meet with the Vietnamese to address their humanitarian concerns. Further, there were three 10-day periods of joint investigations along with a visit by a U.S. forensic team to examine remains unilaterally made available by the Vietnamese.

Throughout 1989, the joint investigation efforts continued in Vietnam, five in all, along with four technical meetings and additional visits by the U.S. forensic team. Concrete results from the joint investigations were disappointing. In another attempt to improve the pace of results, General Vessey again led an Interagency Delegation to Hanoi in October. These discussions resulted in agreements which, if seriously implemented by the Vietnamese, would expedite resolution of the issue.

Activities in 1990 followed along the lines of 1989 with a technical meeting in January followed by two periods of joint investigations in February and May. On September 29, Secretary of State James Baker and Minister Thach met in New York. During the meeting, Secretary Baker stressed the need for rapid POW/MIA progress and agreed to permit Minister Thach and a Vietnamese delegation to travel to Washington, D.C. to meet with General Vessey and the POW/MIA Interagency Group.

On October 17, 1990, a Vietnamese delegation headed by Vietnam's Vice Premier and Minister Thach met in Washington, D.C. with General Vessey and senior U.S. representatives. At this meeting, Minister Thach agreed to all U.S. proposals, to include improved cooperative planning for joint investigations, increased unilateral remains repatriations and serious cooperation to locate and make available wartime documents and records.

Minister Thach also agreed to assist in facilitating access to witnesses to incidents of loss and to military units involved in operations in which U.S. personnel were captured or casualties occurred. He agreed to additional military participation in the joint activities and to allow the U.S. teams to stay on-site until thorough investigations of selected cases are completed.

On April 9, 1991, U.S. policy concerning normalization of relations with Vietnam was presented to Vietnamese Officials in New York. This policy, called the "road map," outlined a series of quid pro quo steps the U.S. was prepared to take to improve U.S.-SRV relations and eventually lead to the normalization of relations.

These measures would include such actions as the gradual lifting of the trade embargo and economic aid. These measures were clearly designed to be implemented only in response to specific Vietnamese actions on POW/MIA and Cambodia settlement-related matters.

On April 19 and 20, 1991, General Vessey again led an Interagency Delegation to Hanoi to meet with Minister Thach and other Vietnamese officials. At these discussions, General Vessey reviewed the progress in implementing steps agreed upon in their October 1990 meeting. Both governments agreed that a temporary POW/MIA office would be established in Hanoi to facilitate rapid resolution of unresolved cases of missing U.S. personnel and provide an administrative and logistics support case for all POW/MIA activities in Vietnam.

The office opened officially on July 8, 1991 with a staff of five. The success of the office led, in part, to the decision to establish the Joint Task Force-Full Accounting within the United States Pacific Command during January 1992.

Subsequent to the opening of the office, General Vessey traveled to Hanoi in October 1991 to meet with Vietnamese Foreign Minister Nguyen

Manh Cam, who had been appointed to replace outgoing Foreign Minister Thach. General Vessey and Foreign Minister Cam reaffirmed the agreements that General Vessey had reached in April 1991 with Minister Thach, emphasizing the need for access to Vietnamese archival records known to be comprehensive.

In February 1992, General Vessey returned to Hanoi to assess progress on POW/MIA matters. During the visit, the Vietnamese provided General Vessey with a long sought-after document of interest to U.S. investigators and analysts concerning Americans shot down in Military Region IV during the Vietnam War. It is believed that similar documents from other military regions would assist U.S. investigators in accounting for Americans.

One month after the Vessey mission, Assistant Secretary of State Richard Solomon led an Interagency Delegation to Hanoi, Vientiane and Phnom Penh. During the meeting in Hanoi, the United States and Vietnam reached five important agreements, which, if fully implemented, will lead to significant results on our POW/MIA concerns.

The Vietnamese agreed to implementation of a short-notice live-sighting investigation mechanism; access by POW/MIA experts to central and regional records, archives and museums; renewed efforts to locate and return the remains of unaccounted for Americans; trilateral POW/MIA cooperation with Laos and Cambodia; and an expanded program of joint field operations over the next two years, including five operations in the next 10 months.

Though results in accounting for missing Americans have been slow, they are measurable. Over the last 18 months, there has been a marked improvement in the level of U.S.-SRV activity, including the establishment of a short-notice live-sighting investigative mechanism, but results have dropped dramatically in terms of accounting. The strengthened agreements reached in Vietnam by Assistant Secretary Solomon, combined with a desire to signal U.S. commitment to improve relations in the context of approved policy, prompted policy officials in Washington to lift certain aspects of the trade embargo with Vietnam including the ban on telecommunications and two other humanitarian-related steps. The other steps were to grant an exception to the economic embargo with Vietnam to permit commercial sales to meet basic human needs and to lift restrictions on projects by non-governmental and non-profit organizations in Vietnam.

What may perhaps turn out to be the most significant advancement in the U.S. government's negotiations with the SRV began developing in September 1992. Through the efforts of an American civilian under contract to the Department of Defense, wartime records from the Vietnam Central Military Museum were passed to the U.S. Officials.

Included in these materials were photographs of American wartime casualties and crash sites. This material clearly documented that the Vietnamese did indeed hold records that could most certainly help resolve the fates of Americans missing from that war.

On October 9, 1992, Vietnam's Ambassador to the United Nations, Trinh Xuan Lang attended a meeting in Washington D.C. with Cheney and acting Secretary of State Lawrence Eagleburger. At this meeting Ambassador Lang was shown a sample of the photographs and was asked to convey to his government our wish for open access to all such material in the hands of the Vietnamese government. Ambassador Lang agreed on behalf of his government to receive a delegation led by General Vessey in Hanoi the following week for discussions on this subject.

On October 18, 1992, General Vessey met in Hanoi with Vietnam's Prime Minister Vo Van Kiet, Defense Minister Doan Khue, Foreign Minister Cam, Vice Foreign Minister Le Mai and several other senior government officials. The result of these meetings is a new agreement for Vietnam to aggressively collect and present to the U.S. government all information, artifacts and remains they have concerning U.S. MIAs.

Complicating this effort is a Vietnamese law which prohibits foreigners from access to SRV government archives. This law protects their classified materials. This obstacle was overcome by the Vietnamese agreement to collect POW/MIA-related materials from all sources and consolidate it in their military museums, thereby providing access to these records by joint U.S.-Vietnamese research teams.

Much work remains to be done before the full magnitude of this new agreement can be assessed. Extensive collection and analytical work will be required. However, both parties are confident that this new effort should significantly accelerate results on POW/MIA issues. In an effort to assist the Vietnamese government with internal political support for its efforts on behalf of the U.S., General Vessey and the delegation agreed to U.S. government humanitarian support for flood victims in Quang Binh Province and other projects.

Laos

Our sustained effort to obtain the cooperations of the Lao government has met with increased success. A visit by the National League of Families in September 1982 was followed by several high-level U.S.–Lao meetings in 1983 and 1984. These discussions resulted in two visits by the JCRC, the first in Laos since 1975.

During the second visit, JCRC and CIL-HI representatives surveyed the requirements to excavate a crash site in southern Laos. After a substantial delay due to Lao government objections to a purported private cross-border foray, an unprecedented joint operation took place in February 1985 in which a U.S.–Lao team conducted a full-scale excavation of a U.S. Air Force AC-130 aircraft shot down near Pakse, Laos.

The team recovered human remains and some personal effects which resulted in accounting for the 13 men missing in the incident. This first excavation was a major step in efforts to develop a sustained pattern of cooperation with the Lao government on the POW/MIA issue. It was conducted with excellent cooperation by Lao officials.

In addition to regular diplomatic dialogue through the U.S. Charge, numerous high-level POW/MIA meetings with the Lao occurred during 1985-1986, including discussions in New York and Vientiane, Laos. In July 1985, Laos agreed in principle to a second excavation during the coming dry season, and in September of that year Lao representatives traveled to Hawaii for an orientation, briefings and consultations with DoD, JCRC and CIL-HI technical personnel.

The following February, a joint excavation was conducted of an AC-130 loss incident that had occurred in March 1972, in Savannakhet Province, southern Laos. The aircraft had a crew of 14 on board and, although this site had obviously been disturbed, a significant quantity of remains and personal effects was recovered. As a result of detailed forensic and anthropological examination by the CIL, nine of the Americans involved in this incident have been accounted for.

During July 1986 policy-level discussions in Vientiane, the Lao agreed to provide written reports on their investigations of several unaccounted for Americans and to consider other unilateral activities. In August 1987, following the Vessey mission to Hanoi, an Interagency delegation met in Vientiane. At this meeting the Lao agreed to expand POW/MIA cooperation and the U.S. government acknowledged the humanitarian problems of Laos, agreeing to address and respond to them when possible and to encourage private humanitarian organizations to increase their efforts as well.

The following year, numerous policy-level discussions were held in Washington, D.C., New York and Vientaine, resulting in increased POW/MIA cooperation. In May and December of 1988, joint surveys and excavations were conducted. Lao government representatives made a December visit to the JCRC and CIL-HI to gain better understanding of the technical process of accounting for POW/MIAs.

In January 1989, a White House-led Interagency Delegation traveled to Vientaine for policy-level discussions with the Lao Foreign Minister and Vice Foreign Minister on POW/MIA and other bilateral issues. The Lao agreed in principle to the need for investigating cases of U.S. personnel last known alive in Lao control and committed to a year-round work plan and excavation of two crash sites.

This was followed by Lao-U.S. consultations in Vientiane during which the work plan and joint recovery operations were discussed. Two joint excavations were subsequently conducted in March and May. In early November, a State Department-led Interagency delegation reached agreement in principle to an expanded joint program of activities for 1990. During the remainder of the year, several successful joint surveys took place.

In February 1990, agreements were reached between the U.S. and Laos to broaden the level and scope of POW/MIA cooperation. Plans included conducting the first joint investigations into cases of Americans known to be alive in Pathet Lao captivity during the war, expanded survey/recovery operations, continuation of the large-scale joint excavations, and agreement in principle to tripartite (Lao/U.S./SRV) cooperation in an effort to resolve incidents of Americans missing in areas of Laos under control of Vietnamese forces at the time of loss. The Lao government's commitment to permit joint activities in areas of Laos not previously open to U.S. officials was important to the broadened cooperation. In 1990, three joint excavations and numerous sit surveys were conducted.

In meetings with Lao ministerial officials during a December 1990 trip to Vientiane, Principal Deputy Assistant Secretary of Defense for International Security Affairs (PDASD/ISA), Carl Ford, emphasized the advances in Lao cooperation on the POW/MIA and counter-narcotics issues. He addressed the possibility for the provision of humanitarian assistance by the DoD based on this progress in U.S.-Lao relations.

Minister of Foreign Affairs Phoun Sipaseut responded positively to Mr. Ford's presentation and reiterated his government's desire to continue to improve cooperation on POW/MIA and counter-narcotics activities.

Although agreed to in the 1990 year-round program, the first investigation into incidents involving Americans last known to be held in Pathet Lao control did not occur until early 1991. During April 1991, PDASD/ISA Ford met in Vientiane with senior Lao officials. The purpose of the meeting was to present to the Lao a significantly expanded POW/MIA program for the remainder of 1991, as well as a U.S. government proposal to address Lao humanitarian concerns. As a result, during 1991 five joint field operations were conducted with the Lao. Activities included further joint investigations of discrepancy cases, small-scale joint surveys and recoveries and joint crash site excavations.

During 1991, and in response to Lao humanitarian concerns, the DoD provided in excess of 100 tons of humanitarian medical supplies and constructed two five-room schools in remote Lao provinces.

In December 1991, a delegation led by Rear Admiral Michael McDevitt, USN, reached agreement on an expanded plan of joint field operations for 1992. Through July 1992, the U.S. and Lao have completed five periods of joint operations, a welcome increase in the pace of activities; however, more time in the field and greater flexibility while there are necessary to maximize results.

Cambodia

The fact that the majority of the 81 Americans unaccounted for in Cambodia were lost in areas controlled by Vietnamese forces combined with the tragic dislocation and chaos inflicted on the Cambodian people by the Khmer Rouge has severely complicated the task of accounting for Americans missing in that country.

In January 1984, officials in Phnom Penh joined the SRV and the Lao Peoples Democratic Republic in issuing an Indochina Foreign Ministers Communique indicating willingness to cooperate with the United States on the POW/MIA issue.

Between February 1984 and July 1986, the United States repeatedly asked the Vietnamese and Lao governments to urge the Phnom Penh regime to resolve the issue of Americans unaccounted for in Cambodia. Similar appeals for intervention were made through international humanitarian channels and the National League of Families; however, no positive response was received.

In September 1987, after receiving case files from the National League of Families on all Americans missing in Cambodia, Premier and Foreign Minister Hun Sen publicly stated that his government had more than 80 remains of Americans. The United States responded by asking an international organization represented in Cambodia to pursue this matter directly with Phnom Penh.

Through subsequent exchanges initiated by Senator Charles Robb and the National League of Families, Phnom Penh agreed in 1990 to accept a U.S. team of forensic specialists to examine 28 remains, and six were repatriated to the U.S. Army CIL-HI, for further study. It now appears that none of the remains are Americans.

U.S. efforts to obtain the cooperation of the Cambodian officials increased during the summer of 1991 with the publication of photographs purported to depict Americans in captivity. The U.S. Deputy Assistant Secretary of State for East Asian and Pacific Affairs met with representatives of Cambodia in Peking and again in Vientaine, Laos to request urgent cooperation in resolving the questions surrounding the photographs.

Following these meetings, an American Technical Delegation visited Phnom Penh seeking to establish a framework for cooperation on American POW/MIA matters and to conduct further investigations on the photos.

In October 1991, the signing of Paris Agreement signaled the beginning of a comprehensive political settlement in Cambodia. This initiative permitted wider access in Cambodia. Joint field operations in Cambodia were undertaken to recover remains believed to be Americans associated with the 1975 Mayaguez incident. This incident occurred off the coast of Cambodia when Khmer Rouge forces captured the U.S. merchant ship Mayaguez and took its crew prisoner. A subsequent rescue attempt not only failed to rescue the crew, but resulted in the loss of several aircraft and American servicemen. Although the crew was later released unharmed, all exchanges with Communist Cambodia were broken off and further exacerbated by the excess of the Khmer Rouge followed by the Vietnamese invasion of Cambodia.

The State of Cambodia government restored contact with the U.S. following the Vietnamese withdrawal from Cambodia. In January 1992, Cambodian officials were hosted by the JCRC and the CIL for briefings on U.S. government efforts to achieve the fullest possible accounting of missing Americans.

As a result of this visit, agreement was reached with Cambodian authorities to permit the use of U.S. helicopters in joint field operations in Cambodia. U.S. helicopters have increased the flexibility and safety of U.S. teams during joint activities with the Cambodians.

In summary, significant strides have been made in recent years. Some Americans, though far too few, have been accounted for and greater results can and must be achieved. Although all involved are frustrated with the pace, the U.S. government is pursuing every available avenue to determine if Americans are still held captive, to account for the missing and repatriate the remains of those who died serving their country.

Southeast Asia POW/MIA Intelligence Activities
—Wartime Intelligence

In the early 1960s, the collection and analysis of information related to POW/MIAs in Indochina was a top priority of the U.S. Intelligence community. The 1964 buildup of U.S. forces in Southeast Asia generated a steady flow of information on captured or missing U.S. servicemen from many sources, especially enemy documents and refugee interrogation reports.

In early 1966, the intelligence community systematically increased its emphasis on POW/MIA intelligence. U.S. activities and organizations worldwide became involved in collecting and analyzing information related to missing Americans in Indochina.

In June 1966, following Hanoi's announcement that captured airmen would be tried for war crimes, collection efforts were intensified even further. The intelligence community established a network of debriefing and interrogation centers in cooperation with local government intelligence agencies in Vietnam and Laos.

These joint endeavors included in-depth debriefings and interrogations of numerous sources to obtain every piece of information held on POW/MIAs. The U.S. government expanded its collection efforts to include worldwide media coverage of POWs, including monitoring Communist radio broadcasts, as well as news film and still photographs.

The DIA, established in late 1961, initially played only a minor role in POW/MIA intelligence collection and analysis. By 1966, DIA's responsibilities had expanded, and by the following year, the Agency assumed chairmanship of the Interagency POW Intelligence Ad Hoc Committee.

In December 1971, DIA commenced chairing the Defense Department's Intelligence Task Force responsible for worldwide POW/MIA intelligence efforts. The Task Force also facilitated POW/MIA-related communications with U.S. government policy makers.

The withdrawal of U.S. forces from Vietnam in 1973 and the fall of Saigon in 1975 greatly hampered the ability of the intelligence community to collect POW/MIA information. These circumstances severely restricted access to key geographic locations and vastly reduced the level and scope of field reporting.

—Expanded Efforts

In 1982, the Reagan Administration's commitment to resolving the POW/MIA issue resulted in a significant upgrade in priority on POW/MIA intelligence collection and analysis. Since that time the U.S. Intelligence community has given top priority to gathering and analyzing data that could relate to Americans missing in Indochina.

Augmented by intelligence assets and resources throughout the world, DIA's Special Office for POW/MIA Affairs expanded fivefold as it became the focal point for all intelligence information relating to the issue.

DIA provides direct support to the development of policy through the POW/MIA Interagency Group and to the JTF-FA. DIA is also responsible for investigation and analysis of live-sighting reports that could relate to missing Americans. The DIA representative to the JTF-FA detachments leads the in-country live-sighting investigations. The representative also analyzes the results of the archival research and advises policy makers on the applications of these findings.

In 1987, DIA established a special intelligence program to collect intelligence information on POW/MIAs. Known as "Stony Beach," the program includes personnel who carry out a broad range of activities to obtain information essential to accounting for POW/MIA cases.

Stony Beach operations are conducted exclusively in support of the POW/MIA issue. The most important aspect of this project was the creation of an intelligence team in Southeast Asia, dedicated to the gathering of POW/MIA-related information from refugees, displaced persons, and other sources throughout Southeast Asia and the Pacific.

As a result of the increasing openness of the Indochinese governments, the conduct of on-scene investigations of live-sighting reports have become an important part of Stony Beach's activities. Stony Beach has grown from an initial staff of 18 to an authorized strength of 27. As part of this expansion, Stony Beach is establishing operating locations in Vietnam, Laos, Cambodia and the Philippines.

POW/MIA Reporting

Since the fall of Saigon in 1975, the Defense Department has received over 15,000 reports originating from Indochinese refugees; 1,610 of these have been determined to be firsthand live-sighting reports of people believed to be Americans. The balance, over 13,500 are classified as "dog tag" reports (7,284), wartime crash and grave site information reports (3,674), or hearsay reports of living Americans (2,829).

Case Analysis

All POW/MIA information is channeled into DIA for analysis. Any reporting that can possibly be correlated to a missing American, regardless of its substance or reliability, is provided to the individual's parent service for prompt transmittal to the next of kin.

Detailed field reports on each case investigated in-country are generated by the investigation and are forwarded to DIA for analysis. The entire investigative process is conducted on the assumption that the individual in question is alive and continues on that basis until clarifying evidence is obtained.

If death is confirmed, investigations and negotiations continue until remains are recovered or convincing evidence is obtained that remains are not likely to be recoverable.

When any information is obtained, it is first compared to data in U.S. files that contain the known facts of the specific case. The information received, usually from local "eyewitnesses," is then evaluated with respect to the plausibility of the account, the consistency and cohesiveness of the narrative, the amount of information provided and the source's creditability.

From this, analysts identify further information requirements and recommend follow-up action, which may include the host government furnishing data from their files. If evidence confirms that the missing serviceman is dead, investigators attempt to acquire absolute proof of death and the possibility of remains recovery is assessed and pursued.

A case is not considered resolved until the man is returned alive, his identifiable remains are repatriated, or the U.S. obtains convincing information as to why neither is possible. In all cases, clear and convincing evidence must be obtained before this judgement is rendered.

Conclusion

Despite the large volume of reports received and the considerable technical means at the disposal of the intelligence community, no single report or combination of reports and technical sensors has thus offered conclusive evidence that any Americans are currently in captivity in Southeast Asia.

The knowledge that some missing Americans initially survived their loss incident and the continued reporting related to potential American POWs, precludes ruling out the possibility that some are still alive in Indochina; therefore, the intelligence community will continue to exert every effort, employ every means, and track down every lead until the fullest possible accounting has been obtained.

"Dog Tag" Reports

Over the past decade, the DoD has received one type of POW/MIA-related report more often than any other. These "dog-tag" reports are accounts in which persons in Vietnam, Laos and Cambodia claim to possess the remains of one or more Americans.

As proof, the sources offer data copied from a dog tag or identification card. In some instances, the source of the report forwards actual metal tags or other indentification materials. Since 1982, the Defense Department has received more than 7,400 such reports.

The names of almost 6,200 American servicemen have been included in this body of dog-tag reporting. Ninety-two percent of those named served with U.S. forces in Southeast Asia and returned alive following their tours of duty. Five percent of the men named were killed in Indochina, their remains recovered, identified, and returned by U. S. forces.

The remaining three percent of the names reported relate to missing Americans.

Although the nature of dog-tag reporting suggests that the remains of personal effects of these servicemen have been recovered by private citizens, follow-up investigation and analysis indicates that this is highly unlikely.

For instance, in the cases of several missing men more than 20 different people claim to have recovered the remains of the same servicemen. Frequently, recovery data and locations differ, suggesting that these people did not obtain their information by the means they claim.

Also, it is not unusual for the same source to be holding more than one set of remains. While a source may name actual missing Americans, at the same time he may also profess to have information on veterans known to be alive in the U.S. Such reports are obviously false.

Generally, the dog-tag reports are forwarded through intermediaries. The information originates with an unnamed person who persuades an acquaintance in one of the Indochinese countries to send it to a relative or friend residing in another country. In this manner many honest people are being induced into conveying information they believe to be true. More recently, with the influx of American tourists in Southeast Asia, it is increasingly common for this type of data to be passed to visitors.

Throughout the war in Southeast Asia, the North Vietnamese had a consistent policy of finding and burying Americans killed in action and sending to central authorities a report of the burial location along with the man's personal effects and identification.

Captured enemy documents indicated that the government of North Vietnam considered this effort to be extremely important to the "political struggle." Presuming that this was done, the present Vietnamese government should have knowledge of most of the missing men whose names have appeared in the dog-tag reports.

Reporting

Since the fall of Saigon in 1975, the Defense Department has received 15,397 reports possibly pertaining to Americans in Southeast Asia. This reporting has steadily increased in the recent years due to a marked increase in refugees leaving Southeast Asia as well as an increase in the presence of American tourists.

As of October 15, 1992, these reports categorized as follows:

- 1,610 Firsthand Live-Sighting Reports—Individual has personally seen what they believed to be an American alive in Southeast Asia.

- 2,829 Hearsay-Sighting Reports—Individual received the report of a live American from a relative or another third party.

- 3,674 Crash/Grave-site Reports—Individual reports to have knowledge of wartime U.S crash/grave site in Southeast Asia. As most of these sites were in remote areas, local villagers were forced to bury the dead on their own or assist the military in the burials of U.S. servicemen killed in combat.

- 7,378 Dog-Tag Reports—These reports usually are from individuals who claim to have the remains of a missing U.S. serviceman and offer as proof the transcribed data from that person's dog tags.

The majority of the 1,610 firsthand live-sighting reports have been resolved. Investigation and analysis of these reports are as follows:

- 1,121 reports (69 percent) were equated to Americans who have been accounted for such as POW returnees, missionaries, or civilians jailed for violations of Vietnamese laws. Forty-three of these reports contained information on wartime sightings correlating to 33 unaccounted for individuals.

- 392 reports (25 percent) have been determined to be fabrications on the part of the source.

The remaining 97 unresolved firsthand live-sighting reports represent the primary focus of DIA analytical and collection efforts:

- 57 (4 percent) pertain to Americans who are described in a captive environment.

- 40 (2 percent) are reported sightings of Americans in a non-captive environment such as working as a truck driver or married and living with a Vietnamese family.

These unresolved reports are under active investigation and analysis to determine whether these individuals are indeed Americans and if so what is their status (American servicemen, expatriates or some other category.)

Joint Task Force-Full Accounting

JTF-FA is the lead DoD agency directly responsible for conducting field operations to assist in accounting for American military and civilian personnel still missing as a result of the Southeast Asian conflict. JTF-FA was established in January 1992 under the operational command of the Commander-in-Chief, U.S. Pacific Command (CINCPAC).

JTF-FA is headquarted at Camp H.M. Smith, Hawaii. Its detachments in Bangkok, Thailand; Hanoi, Vietnam; Vientaine, Laos; and Phnom Penh, Cambodia; consist of command, investigative and administrative staff. At full strength the task force is assigned 150 investigators, analysts, linguists and other specialists representing each of the four military services and DoD civilians.

Upon its creation, JTF-FA assumed the responsibilities of the former JCRC. It was established, in part, as a result of increased commitments by the governments of Vietnam and Laos, and Cambodian officials to cooperate with and expand field operations. These nations are providing increased, though still limited, access to records, files and potential witnesses.

JTF-FA investigators work closely with DIA specialists, particularly when pursuing live-sighting investigations. Interviewers, who are usually fluent linguists, gather information from former and present government officials and Southeast Asian citizens who may possess information about unaccounted for Americans. These investigations are JTF-FA's most urgent priority.

Task force personnel also investigate "discrepancy" cases involving unaccounted for Americans about whom the Indochinese governments should have knowledge.

Discrepancy cases include those in which the circumstances of loss suggest the possibility Americans survived their incident of loss and were possibly captured. The Southeast Asian nations have neither returned these individuals nor their remains.

The commander of JTF-FA, members of his staff, and detachment personnel meet regularly with officials of Vietnam, Laos and Cambodia to exchange POW/MIA information and analyses. They also seek to establish the means for achieving greater results in case resolution. The meetings have proven a successful forum for generating intergovernmental cooperation to conduct joint investigation at selected locations throughout the Indochinese countries.

JTF-FA also conducts operations to excavate reported aircraft crash sites. In these endeavors, the U.S Army CIL-HI plays a key role.

Many of the unaccounted for Americans were pilots or other air crew members who were lost when their aircraft was shot down or crashed. These excavations, which require the same exacting care and patience as archaeological endeavors, seek remains or other material evidence, such as aircraft parts, life support equipment, and personal items. Any evidence discovered is analyzed in an attempt to account for those aboard.

The JTF also performs appropriate honors for repatriating the remains of unaccounted for Americans. Recovered remains are transported to U.S. soil in a dignified manner to honor those who died serving our nation. Then, they are transferred to CIL-HI for analysis in an effort to establish individual identification.

Achieving the fullest possible accounting for Americans still missing from the Vietnam War will continue to require the concerted efforts of all involved agencies. JTF-FA has assumed the central operational role in this effort. Its role is to collect and analyze data, engage in technical discussions with appropriate officials of the Indochinese countries, and conduct field investigations, site excavations and recovery operations.

U.S. Army Central Identification Laboratory, Hawaii

During the Vietnam Conflict, identification of the remains of service members killed in Southeast Asia was the responsibility of the two mortuaries in Vietnam, located in Saigon and Da Nang.

In March 1973, during the withdrawal of U.S. military personnel from Vietnam, the U.S. Army CIL was established at Camp Samae San, Thailand, to assume responsibility for search, recovery, and identification of remains of American service members killed in Southeast Asia during the Vietnam War.

In May 1976, the entire CIL was relocated in Honolulu, Hawaii and is currently a field element of the Casualty and Memorial Affairs Operations Center of the Total Army Personnel Command in Alexandria, Virginia.

The unit has an authorized strength of 125 military and 28 Department of the Army civilians.

After relocation, the mission was expanded as follows:

- Conducts search and recovery operations in the Pacific area for World War II, Korean War, and Vietnam War dead.

- Applies anthropological and other sophisticated scientific techniques in the processing of remains to establish individual identity.

- Accumulates and catalogs information of American and allied personnel listed as missing in action and those declared dead but body not recovered.

- Performs humanitarian missions as directed by competent authority.

- Provides worldwide emergency support to the Army Memorial Affairs Program and, as required, to the Departments of Navy and Air Force for the search, recovery, and identification of remains.

The process of identification begins with the recovery or return of remains. Remains have been received via three avenues: through CIL's own search and recovery missions with the cooperation of host countries; through official turnovers in which a foreign government provides previously recovered remains to the CIL and through other unofficial friendly or refugee sources.

The CIL field search and recovery teams are capable of conducting thorough area searches and excavations at crash and burial sites to recover remains and personal effects. Crash-site recoveries conducted by the search and recovery team often uncover significant information that can aid in the identification process, such as where remains and personal effects were found in relation to major components of an aircraft.

In the past, the CIL has dispatched its search and recovery teams on missions to Laos, Vietnam, Cambodia, Papua New Guinea, New Britain, Melanesia, the Republic of the Philippines, Canada, Korea, and Malaysia.

Receiving remains through official turnovers from the Vietnamese government has been the primary means by which remains have been returned from Indochina. Fifty-nine (including one from the People's Republic of China) such repatriations have occurred since the CIL was established.

Typically, a joint repatriation team, consisting of members of the JTF-FA and the CIL, travels to the foreign country that is returning the remains. The team conducts an appropriate honors ceremony as the remains are placed on a U.S. Air Force aircraft for return to the United States.

After remains are received at the CIL, forensic and other investigative techniques are applied in the processing of the remains to establish, when possible, individual identities. The CIL employs physical forensic anthropologists and odontologists who perform the identification examinations.

Since the remains received by the CIL are frequently fragmented and commingled, the first step in the identification process is to segregate them into separate and unique individuals. After the segregation process is completed, all dental and anthropological findings are documented on a series of charts, forms and special narrative statements.

Anthropological data can be obtained from skeletal remains to determine age, race, sex, muscularity, handedness, height, and indications of injuries the individual may have received or abnormalities which might have existed. The CIL has radiographic, photographic and microscopic equipment to aid in examination and documentation of the skeletal remains.

After the analysis of dental remains is completed by the forensic odontologist, the findings are entered into the Computer Assisted Post-mortem Identification (CAPMI) System. With the CAPMI system, dental information obtained from an unknown set of remains is rapidly sorted against the antemortem dental base, which at CIL-HI consists of the composite antemortem dental records of those missing and unaccounted for from the Vietnam War.

It is important to understand that the purpose of the CAPMI system is not to make identifications, but to increase the efficiency of the investigation team. The system is designed to provide the investigator with a list of possible matches for each set of remains.

It is then up to the forensic odontologist to examine each listed record manually and make a determination as to the degree of certainty of any identification based on dental comparison. The CAPMI system has proven to be an invaluable management tool at the CIL-HI, saving the forensic odontologist countless man-hours that would have been required to make several difficult identifications to date.

Part 6

And I said, "Oh, that I had wings like a dove!
I would fly away and be at rest."

Psalms 55:7

Important Terms and Questions Related to the POW/MIA Issue

Cold War Incidents:

A term used to describe a category of loss incidents which occurred outside of the context of declared hostilities. These incidents include the confrontation between military units of the United States and those of the Eastern Block countries for the period following World War II until the collapse of the Soviet Union.

Joint Field Activities:

Planned field operations jointly staffed by U.S. and host-country personnel. These operations include such activities as investigation and surveys of suspected grave/crash sites, subsequent evacuation of the grave/crash site and the interviewing of witnesses that hopefully can provide information on specific cases.

Khmer Rouge:

(Red Khmers) Leftist Cambodian revolutionary movement whose goal was the overthrow of the Lon Nol Regime in Phnom Penh. Under the leadership of Pol Pot, they succeeded on April 17, 1975, two weeks before the fall of Saigon, when Phnom Penh surrendered to the Khmer Rouge.

In an attempt to transform Cambodia into a totally agrarian society, the Khmer Rouge implemented one of the most radical and brutal restructurings of society ever attempted. They systematically began executing millions of the middle-class citizens and anyone possessing an advanced education.

In 1978, as a result of a series of border disputes, the Vietnamese invaded Cambodia driving the Khmer Rouge from power.

Normalization:

With the collapse of the South Vietnamese government and subsequent Communist takeover in 1975, formal diplomatic relations between Vietnam and the United States were severed.

The term "normalization" refers to the reestablishment of diplomatic channels of communications such as the reopening of embassies and the exchange of ambassadors. In regard to Vietnam, U.S. policy was clearly outlined via a series of quid pro quo steps commonly referred to as the "road map" that would bring the two nations back to pre-1975 status.

Progress on POW/MIA efforts is clearly an essential factor in U.S. government policy concerning normalization.

Pathet Lao:

(Land of the Lao) Vietnamese-supported forces of "liberation" in Laos. Organization had its roots in the original Indochina Communist Party founded by Ho Chi Minh in 1930 and the Vietnamese Worker's Party of the 1950s.

The Pathet Lao received support from the North Vietnamese and assisted the Vietnamese forces along the border where the Vietnamese operated the "Ho Chi Minh Trail." In 1975 the Pathet Lao evolved into the current Lao People's Revolutionary Party.

Rallier:

A term used throughout the Vietnam War for a person who participated in the South Vietnamese program to accept former North Vietnamese/Viet Cong Soldiers and reacclimate them into the South. The literal translation for the Vietnamese program was "Program for return." These individuals were a good source of intelligence.

Road map:

A U.S. government proposal that outlined our expectations of quantifiable Vietnamese actions that would eventually set the stage for normalization of ties with the U.S. This proposal was drafted so as to establish a series of quid pro quo actions that would remove the obstacles to normalization over a 24-month period.

This "road map" is the only official U.S. government document that clearly articulates the necessary steps that need to be taken on POW/MIA matters and other issues before normalization could occur. The "road map" was presented to the Vietnamese in April 1991.

To date the Vietnamese have never formally accepted the "road map," but the U.S. government continues to maintain that it is our stated approach to the normalization of relations.

Technical Meetings:

Non-policy level meetings held between the staffs of the U.S. and the host-country. These talks are centered around technical considerations of the conduct of ongoing or upcoming operations.

Subjects can include discrepancies in a particular case that require the host country to provide more details, size and composition of field teams, details surrounding field operations such as transportation, visas, equipment and associated costs.

These talks are designed to resolve as many preliminary arrangements in advance to maximize field operations when they occur. Technical meetings do not generally result in any negotiated decisions and are generally held to implement agreements reached by policy delegation meetings between the two countries.

Concurrent with the anthropological and dental analyses, the casualty data analysts use existing information to identify casualties which could be associated with the remains. The CIL maintains files on all individuals who are unaccounted for in Southeast Asia. Data from these files is correlated to a map search which narrows the possibilities for potential association.

This "circle search" is done using maps and computerized data to identify known incident or crash sites falling within an established radius of the reported recovery site of the remains in question. The files of all individuals known to be lost in that circle are analyzed for available identifying data.

If no association is made using the CAPMI system, or no dental structures were recovered with a set of remains, the anthropologists and forensic odontologist then compare the files identified by the casualty data analysts through the "circle search" method with the information obtained from the remains.

If no match results from a comparison of the circumstances of the incident of crash and the characteristics of the individuals involved in the incident with determinations made by the forensic specialists, the radius of the circle search is expanded to include additional individuals for comparison until a match is found or exhausted.

If no identification can be supported by these traditional means, though the scientific staff has narrowed the possibilities to a very few, then there are additional sophisticated techniques which can be used with the assistance of the extramural consultants.

These include computer enhancement of radiographs and photographs, superimposition of an antemortem photograph or radiograph or a skull of other skeletal portion, and mitochondrial DNA sequence analysis of skeletal or dental remains.

The latter is an exciting new development in the forensic sciences, and has the potential of allowing CIL-HI to resolve some previously unidentifiable cases. CIL-HI is currently analyzing the results of 23 such cases.

After thorough documentation of the comparison is completed, the CIL presents its professional findings for review by a team of professional consultants, normally consisting of two senior board-certified physical anthropologists and one senior board-certified forensic odontologist.

Identification findings that are concurred with are provided to the next of kin through the parent military service. The next of kin may exercise the option of soliciting a private opinion from an expert of their choosing.

The opinion of the independent expert, if obtained by the next of kin, is returned to the Army's team of professional consultants to be considered before all information is submitted to the Armed Forces Identification Review Board for their final decision to approve or disapprove the CIL's findings.

The Armed Forces Identification Review Board consists of one primary voting member each from the departments of the Army, Navy (or Marine Corps, if applicable) and Air Force as designated by their respective Departments. The members are in the grade of Colonel, Navy Captain, GS-15 or higher.

After the Armed Forces Identification Review Board has approved an identification, the remains depart Hickam AFB, Hawaii, with full military honors, for the Port Mortuary, Travis AFB, California, where they are held pending disposition instructions from the next of kin. If the team of board-certified professional consultants of the Armed Forces Identification Review Board disapproves a CIL recommendation, the case is referred back to the CIL for further review and processing.

Since 1973, the CIL has received nearly 600 remains from Southeast Asia. Of these sets of remains:

- 321 positively identified as missing personnel. This includes the identification of two German missionaries captured by the Vietnamese during the war.

- 271 from Vietnam.

- 47 from Laos.

- Two from China. These were individuals who were lost during the war along the border of China.

- One from Cambodia. This was the remains of a French journalist.

One hundred fifty-one sets of remains are pending identification or are unidentifiable but cannot be excluded as being Americans.

Over 100 remains are those that have been determined to be Southeast Asian Mongoloid or remains that are pending identification but have been determined not to be American.

Eight remains have been determined to be non-human or what is referred to as "CIL Portions." These CIL portions are non-associable portions such as toe bones which have no identification value and preclude even racial determination, small bone fragments or bone dust.

Missing and Unaccounted For Americans From World War II and the Korean War:

Although many years have passed since the conclusion of World War II and the Korean War, the U.S. government has ongoing efforts to determine the fates of Americans missing and unaccounted for while serving their country in these wars.

This includes the recovery and repatriation of remains whenever possible. Approximately 78,750 Americans were unaccounted for from World War II, and there were over 8,100 from the Korean War; however, there are many differences between those wars and the war in Vietnam.

World War II ended in a clear-cut victory; the U.S. had access to the battlefields, so extensive searches could be conducted. Nevertheless, many men were lost and not recovered. Since 1979, more than 115 sets of World War II remains have been recovered from Papua New Guinea and returned to Hawaii for identification.

Additionally, teams have conducted excavations in Panama, Guam, Okinawa, the Solomon Islands and Wake Island, to name a few. As recently as June 1991, the remains of five U.S. personnel were recovered from Papua New Guinea.

In the case of Korea, the United Nations Command Military Armistice Commission (UNCMAC), which represents the 16 nations which joined the South Koreans in the Korean War, has continued to press for the repatriation of the remains of unaccounted for UN servicemen since the termination of hostilities in 1953.

During Operation Little Switch and Big Switch in 1953, a total of 3,748 U.S. POWs (out of a UN total of 13,457) were repatriated. In 1954, the remains of 1,868 U.S. servicemen (out a total of 4,023) were repatriated in Operation Glory. Of these remains, 866 were declared unknown.

However, there are still over 8,100 U.S. servicemen (out of a UN total of over 10,200) who remain unaccounted for. These include servicemen buried in UN cemeteries in North Korea overrun by the Korean People's Army (KPA) and the Chinese People's Volunteers (CPV), those lost or buried at sea, and others simply reported missing.

Also included are 389 personnel (out of a UN total of 2,233) about whom the KPA/CPV should have knowledge. Information gathered from intelligence sources and POW debriefings suggest that these were individuals who were possibly captured, and if deceased, their remains were under KPA/CPV control.

Other than the repatriations in 1953 and 1954, there has been little progress, despite U.S. and UNCMAC efforts to account for those missing servicemen. The UNC has attempted to influence the other side by returning the remains of four CPV soldiers discovered in the Republic of Korea and by returning the bodies of post-war North Korean civilians who had drowned and washed ashore in the South.

The American Ambassador to Czechoslovakia met with Chinese Representatives in Geneva 77 times between 1955 and 1957 on the issue, to no avail. Offers to return the remains of North Korean civilians and soldiers have been rebuffed. Complete information packages on locations of POW camps and UN cemeteries repeatedly have been ignored.

In 1984 in South Korea, the U.S. Army CIL excavated a battle site based on information received from representatives of Project Freedom, an organization which is seeking the recovery of American remains in the Republic of Korea.

However, none of the exhumed remains were determined to be American. In mid-1985, after extensive research into archive material, Army personnel determined that excavation of a different battle site would not be warranted because of previous, well-documented searches by graves registration personnel.

In 1990 and 1991, the North Koreans turned over the remains of five and eleven servicemen, respectfully, through UNCMAC, to U.S. Congressional Delegations. To date, none of these remains have been identified.

Recently, the North Koreans unilaterally, and without preconditions, offered the repatriation of 30 purported U.S. remains through UNCMAC. The remains were repatriated on May 14 and 28, 1992 and are undergoing analysis at CIL-HI in an effort to establish individual identifications. Hopefully, this most recent repatriation is a sign of North Korea's willingness to finally cooperate with UNCMAC in accounting as fully as possible for those unaccounted for from this conflict.

Discussions with the North Koreans on the subject of unaccounted for personnel are conducted by the UNCMAC, which provides updated information to the KPA/CPV MAC as it surfaces. The UNCMAC acts on behalf of all 16 UNC member nations, as well as the Republic of Korea, whose men fought and died in the defense of freedom in Korea. At every opportunity, the U.S. government continues to press for the fullest possible accounting of Americans still missing as a result of the Korean War.

Operation Desert Storm

During the war, a total of 52 American military personnel were listed as missing in action. A number of American journalists were also reported missing in or near enemy-controlled territory. These journalists were all captured and released by the Iraqis. On May 22, 1991, the status of the last American listed as missing in action in Iraq was officially changed to killed in action.

A breakdown of the 52 military personnel listed as missing in or near Iraqi-controlled territories during the war follows:

	Totals	USA	USAF	USN	USMC
Captured & Released	23	7	8	3	5
KIA Body Recovered	26	0	20	3	3
KIA Body Not Recovered	3	0	0	3	0
Missing In Action	0	0	0	0	0
Totals	**52**	**7**	**28**	**9**	**8**

As a result of utilizing the lessons learned from Vietnam and previous wars, the U.S. was successful in accounting for all MIAs from Operation Desert Storm. The establishment of a Joint Rescue Coordination Center prior to the onset of hostilities and the coordination among DIA, the National Prisoner of War Information Center within the DoD, the Service Casualty Officers and other relevant agencies, facilitated immediate efforts to account for all MIAs.

Additionally, improvements in communications technology and a terrain that was less hostile than the jungles of Indochina led to more rapid location and identification of crash sites and remains.

Joint United States—Russian Commission POW/MIAs

In response to demarches presented to the Soviets in April 1991, concerning Americans unaccounted for in the Soviet Union, as well as visits to the Soviet Union by the Senate Select Committee on POW/MIA Affairs and the Under Secretary of Defense for Policy, Paul Wolfowitz, during 1991-1992, the Russian government proposed the formation of a Joint Commission, through which regular bilateral discussions on the subject of American POWs in the former Soviet Union and Russian POWs in the hands of the Afgahanis might be held.

The United States accepted the offer and the United States and Russia inaugurated a Joint Commission on POW/MIAs in Moscow on March 26,

1992. Heading the United States Delegation is former Ambassador to the Soviet Union, Malcom Toon.

The U.S. Commissioners include: Senators John Kerry and Bob Smith, Congressmen Pete Peterson and John Miller; Alan C. Ptak, Deputy Assistant Secretary of Defense (POW/MIA Affairs); A. Denis Clift, Chief of Staff, DIA; Deputy Assistant Secretaries of State Kenneth Quinn, (East Asia and Pacific Affairs) and Richard Kanzlarich, (Canadian and European Affairs); and Dr. Trudy Peterson, Assistant National Archivist. The Russian delegation is led by Colonel General Dimitri Volkogonov, President Boris Yelstin's Senior Military Advisor.

The charter of the Joint Commission encompasses World War II, the Korean War, the Vietnam War and "Cold War" loss incidents. The goals of the Joint Commission are threefold:

- To pursue all reports alleging the presence of American POWs or MIAs in the former Soviet Union, to include assistance in facilitating the return of such individuals if they so wish;

- To establish a mechanism by which remains identified as American can be returned to the United States;

- To obtain access to people, documents and archival information in Russia which could shed light on the fate of unaccounted for American servicemen from World War II, the Korean War, "Cold War" loss incidents, and the Vietnam War.

At the inaugural meeting of the Joint Commission, the two sides established a framework for continued cooperation and follow-on activities to accomplish the agreed upon goals. The two sides discussed specific informational requirements peculiar to each of the categories of losses and toured Russian archives said to contain information pertaining to POW/MIAs.

On May 27, 1992, a working-level U.S. delegation led by DoD Director for POW/MIA Affairs, Ed Ross, who is the commissioner's executive secretary, traveled to Russia to meet with their Russian counterparts to review the Russian progress to date and to discuss ways in which further progress might be achieved.

During this meeting, the Russians provided numerous documents to contain information concerning American servicemen from World War II, Korea and the "Cold War." The materials have been analyzed and some new leads have developed. All materials will be made public at the completion of the commission's work.

The U.S. Army has been designated as executive agent and has established Task Force Russia to oversee investigative and research operations in Moscow. These efforts will include interviewing Russians who may have information on American POWs and research into Russian archives of interest. Task Force Russia has an authorized strength of 40 persons including a Moscow element of 10 individuals.

Following President Yelstin's statement in June 1992 suggesting American POWs may have been taken to the Soviet Union, President Bush directed Ambassador Toon to travel to Moscow to follow-up on the report. The trip uncovered no information to substantiate President Yelstin's claim.

On September 20, 1992, the U.S. Delegation again traveled to Moscow to meet with Russian officials and discuss new initiatives. During this trip Ambassador Toon met with President Yelstin, who reaffirmed his support for the work of the Joint Commission. The delegation also visited a prison camp in eastern Siberia and interviewed Soviet veterans and current officials of Russian Intelligence organizations.

While the establishment of the Commission and the assurances from the Russians that they will provide any information within their records bodes well for the ultimate success of the venture, it remains to be seen whether their performance will live up to their promises.

It is clear, however, that the U.S. government must seize this unprecedented opportunity while it is available and make the most of the information received for the benefit of the affected families.

Frequently Asked Questions

1. **What Is a "Discrepancy Case?"**

   Answer: A discrepancy case is a case about which the U.S. government has convincing evidence that the governments of Vietnam, Laos or Cambodia should have specific knowledge. There are three sub-categories of discrepancy cases: (1) last known alive; (2) listed POW at Homecoming; and (3) all other discrepancy cases in which an Indochinese government should have "specific knowledge of the incident."

   (1) Last Known Alive: Those cases in which the U.S. has information that the individual survived the incident of loss and fell into enemy hands. In the case of air incidents, this includes cases in which the crew members are believed to have successfully exited their aircraft and to have been alive on the ground. In the cases of ground incidents, this includes cases in which the individuals were last known alive, were not gravely wounded, and were in proximity to enemy forces who should have specific knowledge of the incident.

   (2) POW At Homecoming: A specific group of individuals who, during the Vietnam War, were classified by their commanding officers and service secretaries as POWs but did not return during Operation Homecoming

(February-April 1973). These cases are also known to many families as "last known alive" due to their POW status. There were 97 individuals so listed. Subsequently, 42 of these "listed POWs at Homecoming" have been accounted for through unilateral SRV remains repatriations.

(3) Knowledge of the Incident: Circumstances of loss or subsequent information is convincing that Vietnam, Laos or Cambodia should have knowledge of the incident. In some of these cases, there is convincing evidence that the individual did not survive the incident of loss. In many cases, there is convincing evidence that Vietnam also has remains.

2. **Why Has the U.S. Government Not Placed All of the Individuals on the List of Unaccounted For Who Participated in the "Secret War" in Laos or Who Participated in So Called "Black Operations" in Southeast Asia?**
Answer: The list of unaccounted for Americans from the Vietnam War is complete. All individuals, including CIA agents and others involved in sensitive or clandestine operations in Southeast Asia, have been incorporated into the list of 2,267 Americans who are unaccounted for. There is no "secret list" and the U.S. government is actively engaged in the task of achieving the fullest possible accounting for these missing Americans.

3. **Why Is POW/MIA Information Classified So That Even the Families Are Not Permitted To See It?**
Answer: As a matter of U.S. government policy since 1982 and pursuant to federal law since 1988, the DoD provides to the primary next of kin (PNOK) copies of all reports which correlate or may correlate to their loved one. Where information in the reports is classified, the report must be declassified before it may be released to the family.

The only information deleted from the classified report is information, which, if disclosed, would harm ongoing and future U.S. government efforts to account for missing Americans. The declassified reports are then forwarded to the PNOK through the respective Service Casualty Officer.

The DoD has also begun the process of collection, collation, processing, and, as appropriate, declassification of DoD records on Vietnam Era POW/MIAs consistent with the provisions of Section 1082 of the National Defense Authorization Act for Fiscal Years 1992 and 1993. A DoD Central Documentation Office has been established to carry out these tasks and military personnel and civilians have been at work on the project since February 1992.

Under new Classification Guidance issued in February 1992 by the Assistant Secretary of Defense for Command, Control, Communications and

Intelligence, information including "live-sighting reports" will be declassified following investigation and analysis.

After the investigation is completed and the conclusions approved by an interagency panel of intelligence experts, the reports will be furnished to the Central Documentation Office for declassification. Previously, live-sighting reports remained classified after the investigation had been concluded.

Section 1082 of the National Defense Authorization Act requires that information concerning Americans unaccounted for from the Vietnam War be made public, subject to the approval of the PNOK of the individual involved.

The information approved by PNOK for release will be placed in a special reading room at the Library of Congress so that it may be accessed by the general public. For those not in the Washington, D.C. area, this information can be accessed through the Inter Library Service.

President Bush issued Executive Order 12812 on July 22, 1992, directing that all classified documents from the Vietnam era dealing with POW/MIA matters be declassified and made available to the American public.

All material is included under this executive order with the exception of material that would jeopardize ongoing U.S. government efforts or compromise sensitive intelligence sources or methods. To date, 100,500 pages have been declassified and released.

When completed in the summer of 1993, nearly 1.5 million pages of documents will have been made available. This material is available to the public on microfiche through their local library of Congress lending program.

4. Isn't It True That the Vietnamese Held Back French POWs After the French Indochina War, and Therefore We Should Expect That U.S. POWs Would Also Be Retained Following the Paris Peace Agreement?
Answer: In 1954, 6,900 persons including 2,200 ethnic French, were carried as missing from the French expeditionary forces. These were not prisoners, but rather individuals who were lost under uncertain conditions.

All French prisoners were returned by the end of 1954. A small number of non-French and non-Vietnamese remained in North Vietnam, but not against their will. Of the Vietnamese serving in French forces who were carried as missing, some had "rallied" to the other side before the Geneva Accords. According to the French government, the Geneva Accords were implemented, and no one remained against his will.

5. Is It True That the Department Of Defense Has Provided Empty Caskets To Families For Burial?
Answer: The DoD has never provided to a family an empty coffin for burial. In cases where several individuals perished in the same incident and the remains of the individuals can be individually segregated, the PNOK of the individuals are provided the opportunity to decide whether they desire that their loved one's remains be interred separately or as part of a group burial. Where the remains cannot be individually segregated, but it can be forensically established that the number of remains represented is equal to the number of persons in the incident, the remains are interred in a group burial with the names of all the individuals on the marker.

Where it cannot be forensically established that the remains equal the number of persons in the incident, but the evidence establishes that no one survived the incident of loss, the remains are interred as a group and, with the approval of the PNOK, the names of all of the individuals are placed on the marker.

6. Why Do You Spend Your Time "Digging Up Bones" In Southeast Asia Rather Than Concentrating On Finding Live Americans?
Answer: The most urgent priority of U.S. government POW/MIA efforts is to determine whether Americans are alive in Southeast Asia and, if so, return them to the United States. Until the past year, we have been unable to investigate "live-sighting" reports on short notice due to decisions by the governments in Indochina. Such decisions must be respected as matters of the individual nation's sovereignty. In the past several months, DoD investigators have been permitted to conduct live-sighting investigations on short notice in Vietnam and Cambodia. Although Laos has not yet agreed to this important aspect of our efforts, the government of Laos did provide excellent cooperation in successfully investigating highly visible photographs which were determined not to be U.S. personnel.

Because our first priority is to determine whether Americans may still be held in Southeast Asia, we have identified a category of individual cases wherein the individual is believed to have survived his incident of loss and been in close proximity to enemy forces and likely to have been captured, or for whom the Vietnamese, Laotians or Cambodians should be able to account.

We believe the greatest possibility of finding a live American POW, based upon the individual circumstances of loss, is among the last known live cases; however, several hundred Americans were lost under circumstances which are still unknown to the U.S. government and the possibility of their survival can be excluded.

To investigate the last known alive cases, we conduct live-sighting investigations, joint field investigations in the three Indochina countries, and lastly, the excavation of crash sites and grave sites when evidence confirms that the individual is dead. Our investigators have no preconceived notions of fate and go where the evidence takes them. If the evidence confirms death, we attempt to recover and identify remains to fully resolve the family's uncertainty.

Location and recovery of the remains of the last known alive category of individuals sheds important light on the live-prisoner issue. Efforts to investigate live-sightings, conduct joint field investigations, and finally, excavation and recovery of remains, are inextricably-related complimentary parts of the process of resolving the live-prisoner issue and achieving the fullest possible accounting.

Part 7

The Lord is near to the broken hearted and will save those whose spirits are crushed.

Psalms 34:18

POW/MIA Photos

There are not many towns in the United States where the people can honestly say they wholeheartedly welcomed a Vietnam veteran home after the war. In most towns in America, at least one of its young soldiers was killed in the war. Many towns had some who never returned because of being a Prisoner of War or Missing in Action. Almost all towns had some veterans come home with no welcome.

When my Father returned home from World War II, he had no parade, no reunion, no anything. But . . . he had a Nation behind him and he knew it and was very proud for what he had done. Not only did many Vietnam veterans not have the nation behind them, they did not even have their families behind them.

In my hometown, we lost two of our finest young men in the fighting in Vietnam. Two others, Allan Newman and Wayne Porter, returned home safely, but, with the typical "no welcome home." Looking back now, it is exactly what hundreds of thousands of other Vietnam veterans faced upon their return. I had watched all four of these fine young men graduate from high school. I know their families personally and they are the cream of the crop.

Allan had served with the U.S. Marines and Wayne was a helicopter pilot with the 1st. Cavalry. I called Wayne recently and told him that he would probably think I was crazy, but I apologized for not welcoming him home from the War. I told him I was sorry for not visiting with him to talk about his time in Vietnam.

He was quiet for a moment then said, "Well, 20 years is an awful long time but . . . you are still the first." Nothing made me feel better than that phone call.

As a veteran and an American, I know that in the face of silence, indifference and hostility, the United States abandoned some of the men it sent into battle. And, as a veteran and an American, I will not rest until I am certain it will never happen again.

We can call the families of the POW/MIAs and tell them that they, and their loved ones, are on our hearts and in our prayers. We can tell them we will never rest until we are certain that there has been a full accounting of all American POW/MIAs. We can continue asking our government to press Vietnam, Laos, Cambodia, China and Russia for answers about our POW/MIAs, America's Missing Men.

Chimp Robertson
Tahlequah, Oklahoma

Dear Chimp:

To help resolve the unanswered questions concerning the nation's POW/MIAs from Southeast Asia, I voted in favor of the McCain-Kerry amendment to the Department of State Re-authorization legislation urging the President to lift the embargo against Vietnam. The Senate passed the amendment on January 27, 1994, by a vote of 68 to 32. President Clinton announced the lifting of the U.S. trade embargo against Vietnam on February 3, 1994.

The McCain-Kerry amendment was not about rewarding Vietnam or trusting Vietnam. The vote was a judgment about the best way to achieve our nation's goals and serve the interests of our unaccounted-for and their families. Americans currently in Vietnam conducting the search for the missing agree that lifting the embargo not only will facilitate the effort, but is necessary for its continuance and successful conclusion. If this is the tool they request, we should provide it for them.

Furthermore, I was impressed by the fact that all of the members of the Senate who are combat veterans from Vietnam supported the McCain-Kerry amendment.

Previously (August 1991), I co-sponsored a resolution which created the Senate Select Committee on POW/MIA Affairs. The Select Committee was created to fulfill a national obligation to personnel still listed as unaccounted-for in Southeast Asia and to their families. The Select Committee held 22 days of public hearings which incorporated testimony from 144 witnesses, including former Secretaries of Defense and State, former North Vietnamese military officials, and members of POW families and advocacy groups.

The Select Committee on POW/MIA Affairs concluded its work in January 1993, by submitting its findings to Congress. The Select Committee stated in its report, "There is . . . no compelling evidence that proves that any American remains alive in captivity in Southeast Asia." However, while the Committee acknowledged that there is no proof that all who remained in Southeast Asia have died, the Committee agreed that it is essential to continue efforts toward the fullest possible accounting of our missing Americans.

The Select Committee's authorization expired on January 3, 1993, but further work has been achieved by the Joint Task Force-Full Accounting. In 1993, 67 remains were repatriated to the United States from Vietnam.

I am determined to do whatever is necessary to resolve the question of our POW/MIA missing in Southeast Asia. I am also committed to honoring these brave Americans. I will continue to support legislation to achieve these goals.

Sincerely,
Carl Levin
United States Senator—Michigan

The photos of POWs in the following section were made available by Mr. Ken Carter of the Department of Defense, Washington, D.C. They are a representative grouping—by no means exhaustive. (My apologies for either the inclusion or non-inclusion of any single POW. An exhaustive portfolio is not possible in a book of this type.)

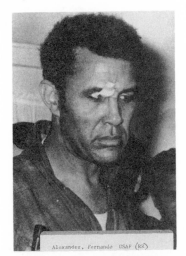

Alexander, Fernando USAF (RR)

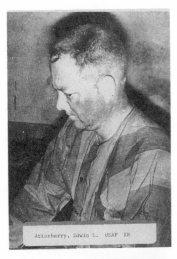

Atterberry, Edwin L. USAF KR

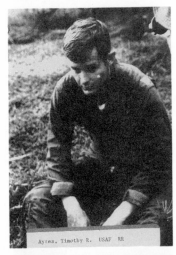

Ayres, Timothy R. USAF RR

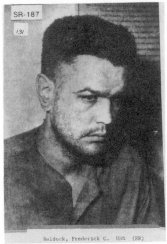

SR-187

131

Baldock, Frederick C. USN (RR)

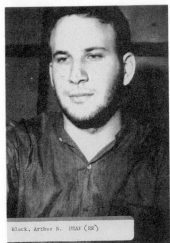

Black, Arthur N. USAF (RR)

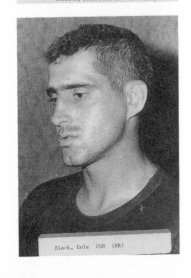

Black, Cole USN (RR)

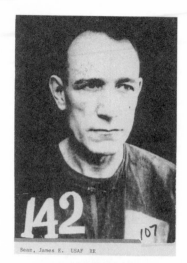

Bean, James E. USAF RR

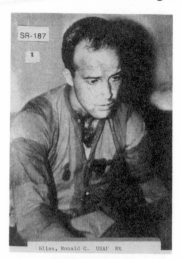

Bliss, Ronald G. USAF RR

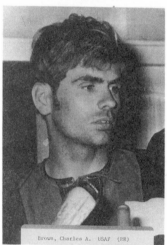

Brown, Charles A. USAF (RR)

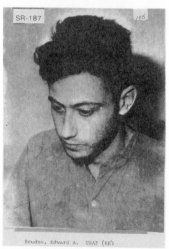

Brudno, Edward A. USAF (RR)

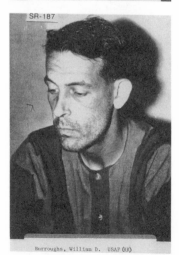

Burroughs, William D. USAF (RR)

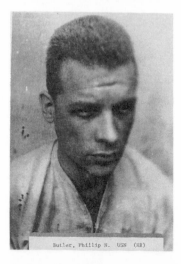

Butler, Phillip N. USN (RR)

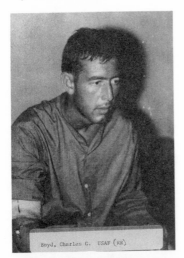

Boyd, Charles G. USAF (RR)

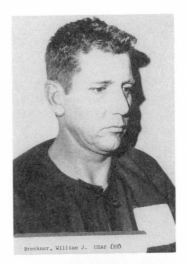

Breckner, William J. USAF (RR)

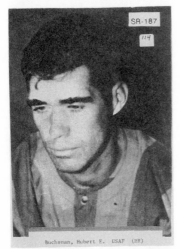

Buchanan, Hubert E. USAF (RR)

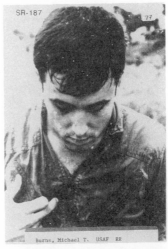

Burns, Michael T. USAF RR

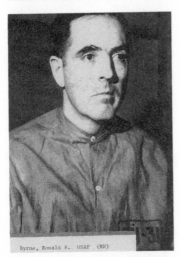

Byrne, Ronald E. USAF (RR)

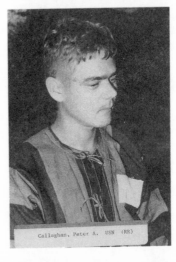

Callaghan, Peter A. USN (RR)

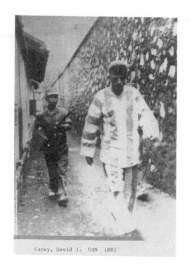

Carey, David J. USN (RR)

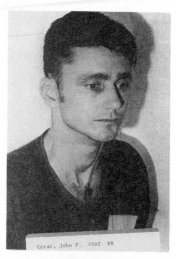

Cerak, John P. USAF RR

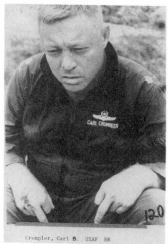

Crumpler, Carl B. USAF RR

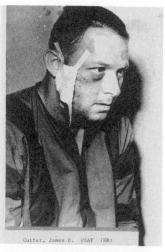

Cutter, James D. USAF (RR)

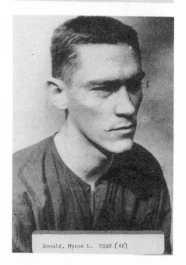

Donald, Myron L. USAF (RR)

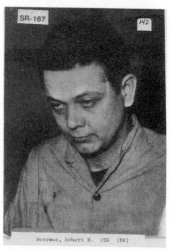

Doremus, Robert H. USN (RR)

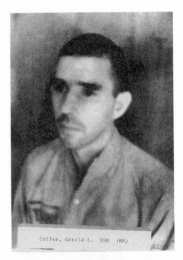

Coffee, Gerald L. USN (RR)

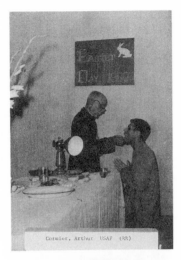

Cormier, Arthur USAF (RR)

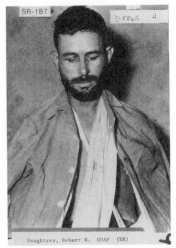

Daughtrey, Robert N. USAF (RR)

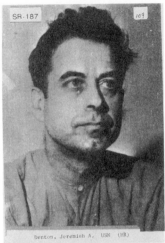

Denton, Jeremiah A. USN (RR)

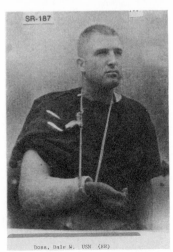

Doss, Dale W. USN (RR)

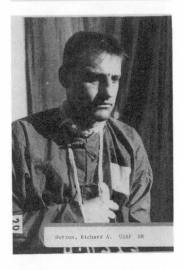

Dutton, Richard A. USAF RR

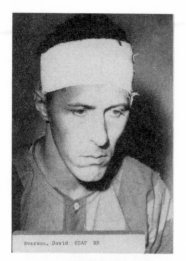

Everson, David USAF RR

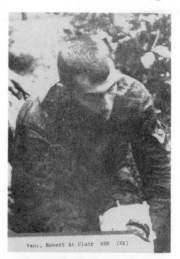

Fant, Robert St Clair USN (RR)

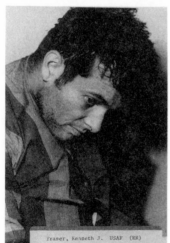

Fraser, Kenneth J. USAF (RR)

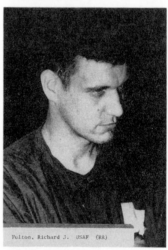

Fulton, Richard J. USAF (RR)

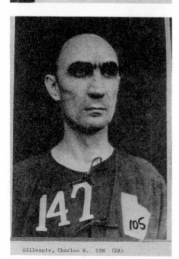

Gillespie, Charles R. USN (RR)

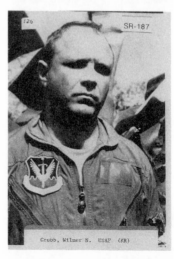

Grubb, Wilmer N. USAF (RR)

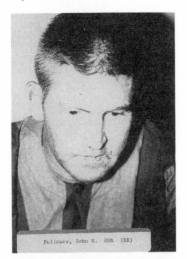

Fellowes, John H. USN (RR)

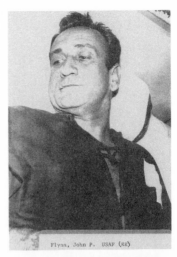

Flynn, John P. USAF (RR)

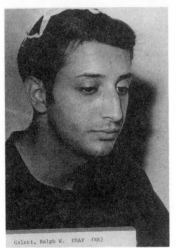

Galati, Ralph W. USAF (RR)

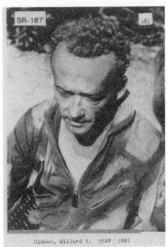

SR-187

Gideon, Willard S. USAF (RR)

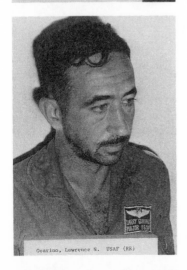

Guarino, Lawrence N. USAF (RR)

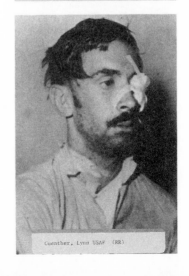

Guenther, Lynn USAF (RR)

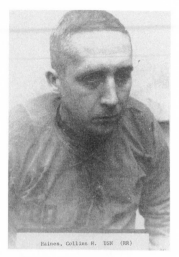

Haines, Collins H. USN (RR)

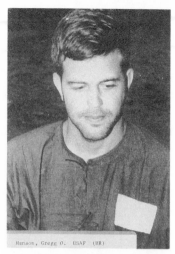

Hanson, Gregg O. USAF (RR)

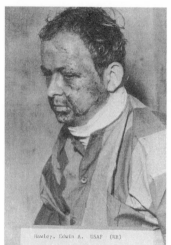

Hawley, Edwin A. USAF (RR)

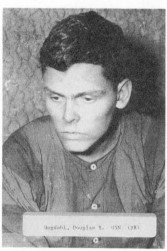

Hegdahl, Douglas B. USN (RR)

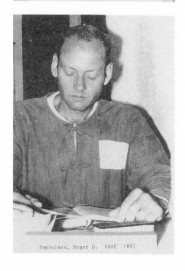

Ingvalson, Roger D. USAF (RR)

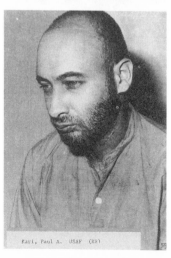

Kari, Paul A. USAF (RR)

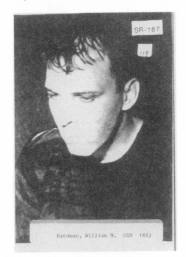

Hardman, William M. USN (RR)

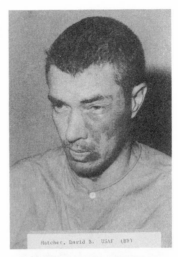

Hatcher, David B. USAF (RR)

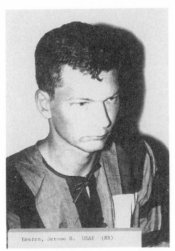

Heeren, Jerome D. USAF (RR)

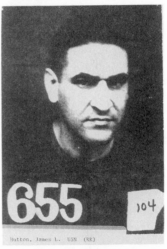

Hutton, James L. USN (RR)

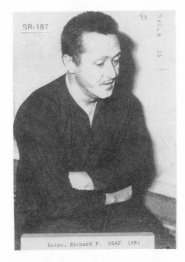

Keirn, Richard P. USAF (RR)

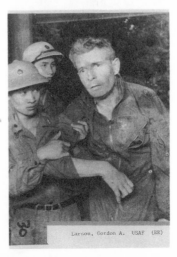

Larson, Gordon A. USAF (RR)

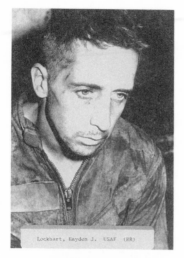

Lockhart, Hayden J. USAF (RR)

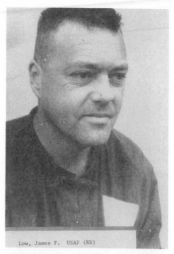

Low, James F. USAF (RR)

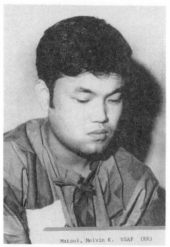

Matsui, Melvin K. USAF (RR)

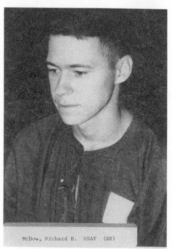

McDow, Richard H. USAF (RR)

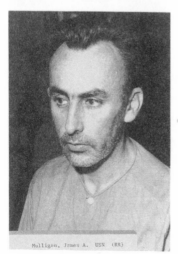

Mulligan, James A. USN (RR)

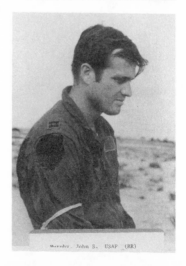

Murphy, John S. USAF (RR)

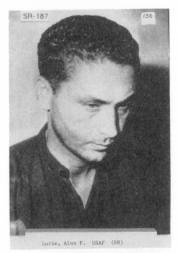

SR-187   156

Lurie, Alan P. USAF (RR)

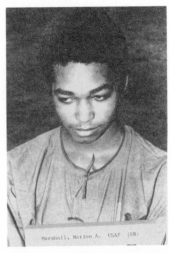

Marshall, Marion A. USAF (RR)

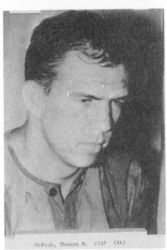

McNish, Thomas M. USAF (RR)

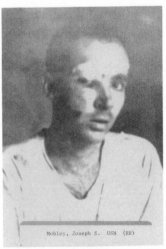

Mobley, Joseph S. USN (RR)

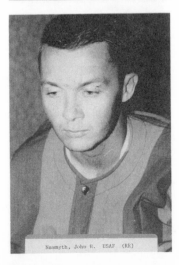

Nasmyth, John H. USAF (RR)

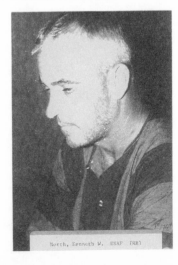

North, Kenneth W. USAF (RR)

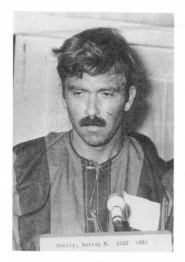

Overly, Norris M. USAF (RR)

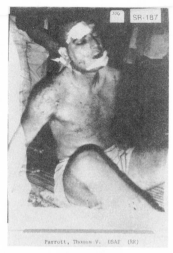

Parrott, Thomas V. USAF (RR)

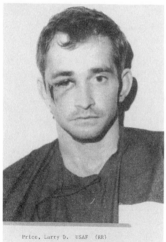

Price, Larry D. USAF (RR)

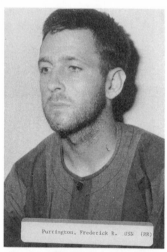

Purrington, Frederick R. USN (RR)

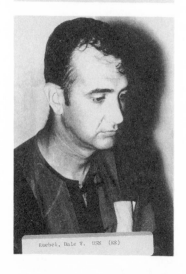

Raebel, Dale V. USN (RR)

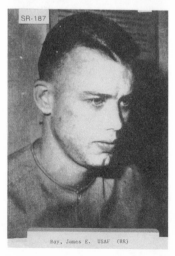

Ray, James E. USAF (RR)

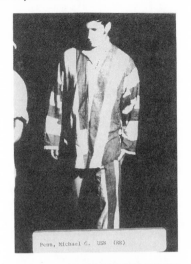

Penn, Michael G. USN (RR)

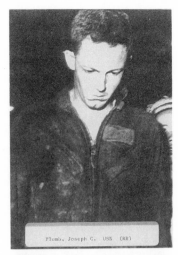

Plumb, Joseph C. USN (RR)

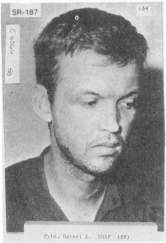

Pyle, Darrel E. USAF (RR)

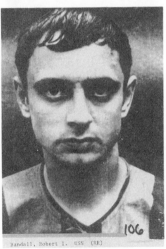

Randall, Robert I. USN (RR)

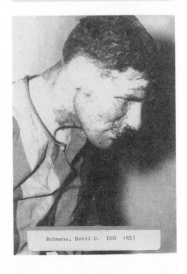

Rehmann, David G. USN (RR)

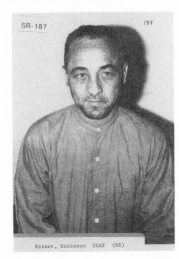

Risner, Robinson USAF (RR)

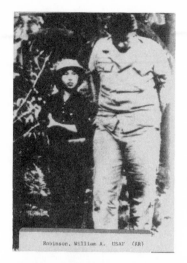

Robinson, William A. USAF (RR)

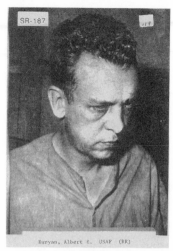

Runyan, Albert E. USAF (RR)

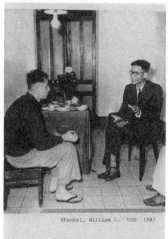

Shankel, William L. USN (RR)

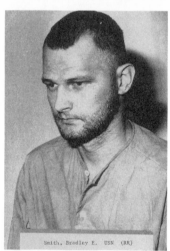

Smith, Bradley E. USN (RR)

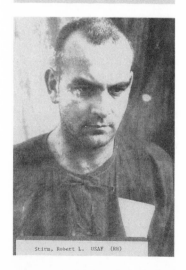

Stirm, Robert L. USAF (RR)

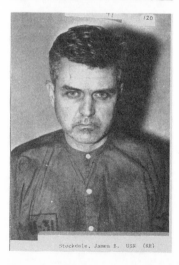

Stockdale, James B. USN (RR)

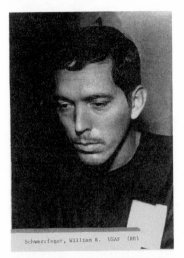

Schwertfeger, William R. USAF (RR)

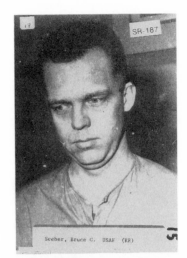

Seeber, Bruce G. USAF (RR)

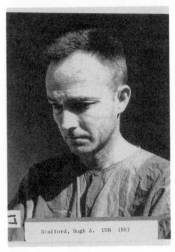

Stafford, Hugh A. USN (RR)

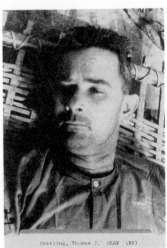

Sterling, Thomas J. USAF (RR)

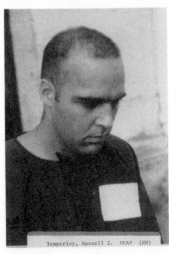

Temperley, Russell E. USAF (RR)

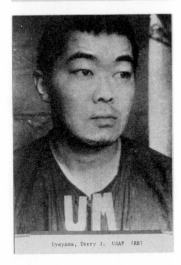

Uyeyama, Terry J. USAF (RR)

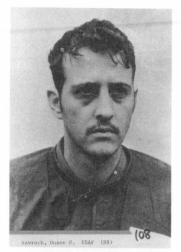

Vavroch, Duane P. USAF (RR)

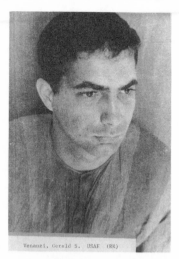

Venanzi, Gerald S. USAF (RR)

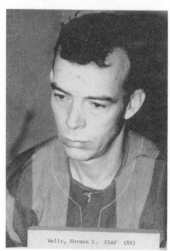

Wells, Norman L. USAF (RR)

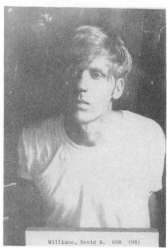

Williams, David B. USN (NR)

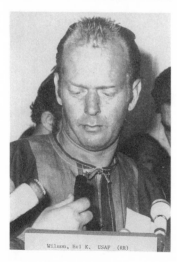

Wilson, Hal K. USAF (RR)

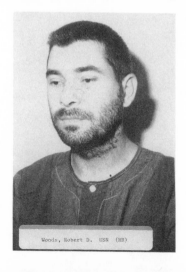

Woods, Robert D. USN (RR)

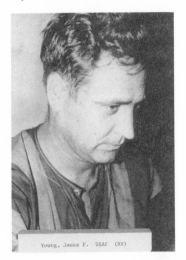

Young, James F. USAF (RR)

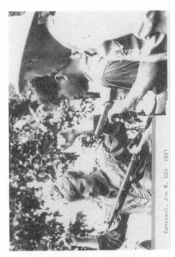

Cleveland, Jon R. USA (RR)

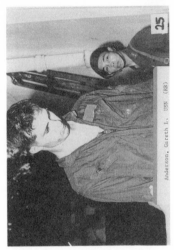

Anderson, Gareth L. USN (RR)

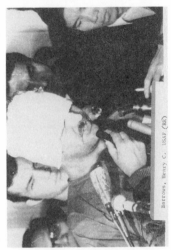

Barrows, Henry C. USAF (RR)

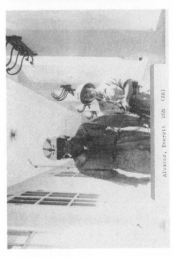

Alvarez, Everett USN (RR)

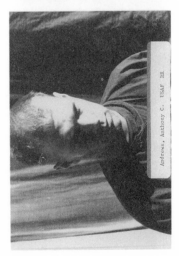

Andrews, Anthony C. USAF RR

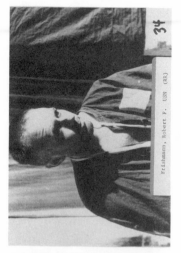

Frishmann, Robert F. USN (RR)

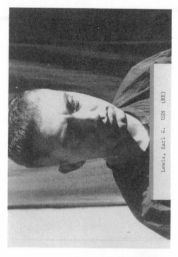

Lewis, Earl G. USN (RR)

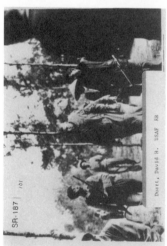

Duart, David R. USAF RR

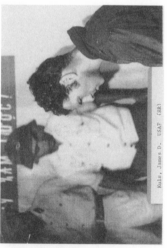

Kula, James D. USAF (RR)

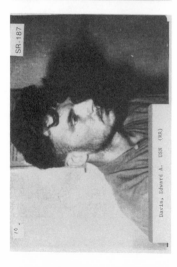

Davis, Edward A. USN (RR)

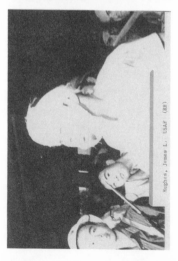

Hughes, James L. USAF (RR)

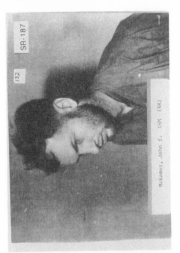

McKamey, John E. USN (RR)

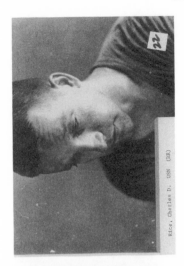

Rice, Charles D. USN (RR)

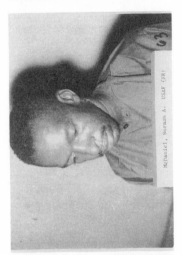

McDaniel, Norman A. USAF (RR)

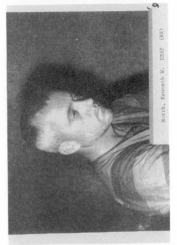

North, Kenneth W. USAF (RR)

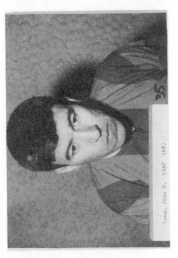

Luna, Jose D. USAF (RR)

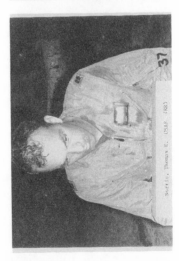

North, Thomas E. (USAF (RR)

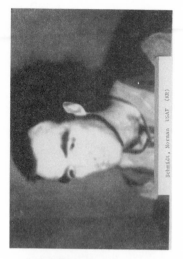

Schmidt, Norman USAF (KR)

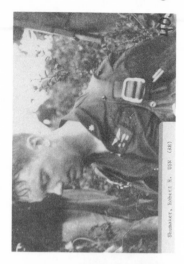

Shumaker, Robert H. USN (RR)

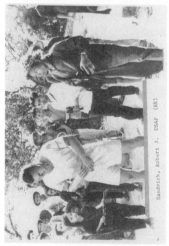

Sandvick, Robert J. USAF (KR)

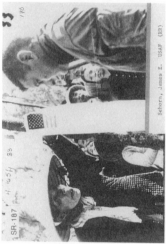

Sehorn, James E. USAF (RR)

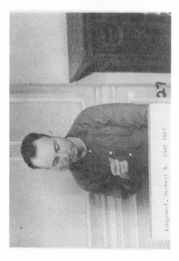

Ringsdorf, Herbert R. USAF (KR)

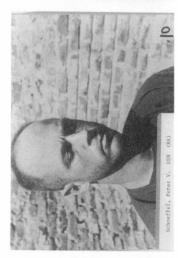

Schoeffel, Peter V. USN (RR)

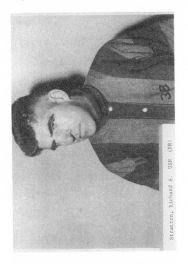

Stratton, Richard A. USN (RR)

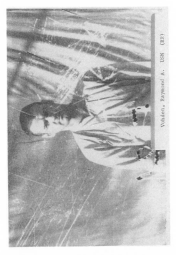

Vohden, Raymond A. USN (RR)

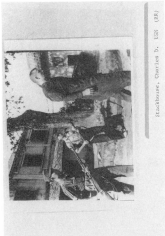

Stockhouse, Charles D. USN (RR)

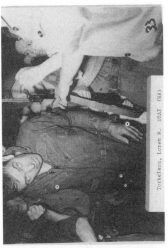

Torkelson, Loren H. USAF (RR)

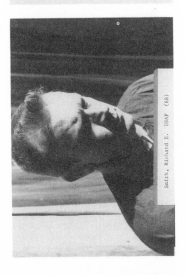

Smith, Richard E. USAF (RR)

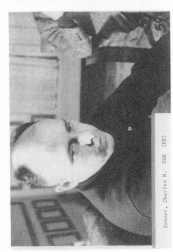

Tanner, Charles N. USN (RR)

Other Books by Starburst Publishers

POW/MIA–America's Missing Men   —Chimp Robertson

Subtitled: *The Men We Left Behind.* Raises questions and relays the thoughts and feelings of more than 75 soldiers, ex-soldiers, senators, congressmen, entertainers and media members about the POW/MIA issue on whether America left its soldiers in Southeast Asia. Quotes and comments include those from: Gen. William C. West-moreland, Senator John Kerry, Oliver North, American Legion Magazine, and the National League of Families of Missing Americans.

(hardcover) ISBN 0914984640   **$19.95**

Nightmare In Dallas   —Beverly Oliver

The hard-hitting account of the mysterious "Babushka Lady," Beverly Oliver, who at the age of seventeen was an eyewitness to the assassination of President John F. Kennedy. This is only the second book to be written by one who saw the event first-hand. Beverly was a personal friend of Jack Ruby and was married to a member of the Mafia. Beverly's film of the event (the only other known motion picture) was confiscated by two men who called themselves FBI agents. To this present day, neither she nor any other known person has been permitted to view the film. Why? This book tells the story.

(hardcover) ISBN 0914984608   **$19.95**

Common Sense Management & Motivation—Roy H. Holmes

Teaches the principles of motivating subordinate personnel via good human relations, It is written from practical "how-to" experience rather than classroom theory. Specific subjects covered include: Basic motivation psychology, Effective communication, Delegating, Goal-setting, Confronting, and Leadership qualities. A must book for all existing or aspiring supervisors, managers, business leaders, and anyone else interested in managing and motivating people.

(hardcover) ISBN 0914984497   **$16.95**

Lease–Purchase America!   —John Ross

A first-of-its-kind book that provides a simple "nuts and bolts" approach to acquiring real estate. Explains how the lease-purchase technique pioneered by John Ross can now be used in real estate to more easily buy and sell a home. Details the value of John's technique from the perspective of each participant in the real estate transaction. Illustrates how the reader can use lease-purchase successfully as a tool to achieve his or her real estate goals.

(trade paper) ISBN 0914984454   **$9.95**

Books by Starburst Publishers—cont'd.

Winning At Golf
David A. Smith

Addresses the growing needs of aspiring young golfers yearning for correct instruction, positive guidance, and discipline. It is an attempt not only to increase the reader's knowledge of the swing, but also sets forth to inspire and motivate the reader to a new and rewarding way of life. **Winning At Golf** relays the teachings of Buck White, the author's mentor and a tour winner many times over. It gives instruction to the serious golfer and challenges the average golfer to excel.

(trade paper) ISBN 0914984462 **$9.95**

The New American Family
—Artlip, Artlip, & Saltzman

American men and women are remarrying at an astounding rate, and nearly 60% of the remarriages involve children under the age of eighteen. Unfortunately, over half of these remarriages also end in divorce, with half of the "redivorces" occuring within five years. **The New American Family** tells it like it is. It gives examples and personal experiences that help you to see that the second time around is no picnic. It provides practical, good-sense suggestions and guidelines for making your new American family the one you always dreamed of.

(trade paper) ISBN 0914984446 **$10.95**

Parenting With Respect and Peacefulness—Louise A. Dietzel

Subtitled: *The Most Difficult Job in the World*. Parents who love and respect themselves parent with respect and peacefulness. Yet, parenting with respect is the most difficult job in the world. This book informs parents that respect and peace communicate love—creating an atmosphere for children to maximize their development as they feel loved, valued, and safe. Parents can learn authority and control by commonsense, interpersonal, and practical approaches to day-to-day issues and situations in parenting.

(trade paper) ISBN 0914984667 **$10.95**

Dr. Kaplan's Lifestyle of the Fit & Famous—Eric Scott Kaplan

Subtitled: *A Wellness Approach to "Thinning and Winning."* A comprehensive guide to the formulas and principles of: FAT LOSS, EXERCISE, VITAMINS, NATURAL HEALTH, SUCCESS and HAPPINESS. More than a health book—it is a lifestyle based on the empirical formulas of healthy living. Dr. Kaplan's food-combining principles take into account all the major food sources (fats, proteins, carbohydrates, sugars, etc.) that when combined within the proper formula (e.g. proteins cannot be mixed with refined carbohydrates) will increase metabolism and decrease the waistline. This allows you to eat the foods you want, feel great, and eliminate craving and binging.

(hardcover) ISBN 091498456X **$21.95**

Stay Well Without Going Broke —Gulling, Renner, & Vargas

Subtitled: *Winning the War Over Medical Bills.* Provides a blueprint for how health care consumers can take more responsibility for monitoring their own health and the cost of its care—a crucial cornerstone of the health care reform movement today. Contains inside information from doctors, pharmacists and hospital personnel on how to get cost-effective care without sacrificing quality. Offers legal strategies to protect your rights when illness is terminal.

(hardcover) ISBN 0914984527 **$22.95**

Migraine –Winning the Fight of Your Life —Charles Theisler

This book describes the hurt, loneliness and agony that migraine sufferers experience and the difficulty they must live with. It explains to the reader the different types of migraines and their symptoms, as well as explaining the related health hazards. Gives 200 ways to help fight off migraines, and shows how to experience fewer headaches, reduce their duration, and decrease the agony and pain involved.

(trade paper) ISBN 0914984632 **$9.95**

Purchasing Information

Listed books are available from your favorite Bookstore, either from current stock or special order. To assist bookstore in locating your selection be sure to give title, author, and ISBN #. If unable to purchase from the bookstore you may order direct from STARBURST PUBLISHERS. When ordering enclose full payment plus $2.50 for shipping and handling ($3.00 if Canada or Overseas). Payment in US Funds only. Please allow two to three weeks minimum (longer overseas) for delivery. Make checks payable to and mail to STARBURST PUBLISHERS, P.O. Box 4123, LANCASTER, PA 17604. Credit card orders may also be placed by calling 1-800-441-1456 (credit card orders only), Mon-Fri, 8 AM-5 PM Eastern Time. **Prices subject to change without notice.**   7-95